Women and Nutrition
in Third World Countries

Women and Nutrition
in Third World Countries

Sahni Hamilton
Barry Popkin
Deborah Spicer

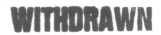

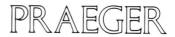

PRAEGER

PRAEGER SPECIAL STUDIES • PRAEGER SCIENTIFIC

New York • Philadelphia • Eastbourne, UK
Toronto • Hong Kong • Tokyo • Sydney

BERGIN & GARVEY PUBLISHERS, INC.

Library of Congress Cataloging in Publication Data

Hamilton, Sahni.
   Women and nutrition in Third World countries.

   Bibliography: p. 115
   Includes index.
   1. Women—Health and hygiene—Developing countries. 2. Women—
Developing countries—Nutrition.   3. Mothers—Developing countries—
Nutrition.   4. Malnutrition in pregnancy—Developing countries.
5. Women—Diseases—Developing countries—Nutritional aspects.
I. Popkin, Barry M.   II. Spicer, Deborah.   III. Title.
RA778.H195   1984   362.1'9639'09172'4   83-25690
ISBN 0-03-000842-5

Published in 1984 by Praeger Publishers
CBS Educational and Professional Publishing
A Division of CBS, Inc.
521 Fifth Avenue, New York, New York 10175 U.S.A.

456789   056   987654321

Printed in the United States of America

Contents

Tables and Figures

Tables

Figures

Preface

Our multidisciplinary research group at the Carolina Population Center has developed an approach over the last three years for addressing problems of nutrition, health, and population in which we attempt to integrate social science research. Focusing on household and community-level issues, we have tried to understand the problems and constraints households face in meeting their health and nutrition needs. Our primary focus has been on infant feeding in low-income countries and the United States, particularly in developing methodologies for analyzing patterns and determinants of breast-feeding and infant supplementary feeding.

We initially studied the adequacy of infant diets because we felt this was one of the major nutrition policy issues facing low-income countries, and one for which more rigorous methodologies for analyzing population-based data were needed. In the process of undertaking research in this area, we found that women were not only at the center of most household decisions affecting infants, but that they faced tremendous economic, time, and sociocultural constraints in meeting household and their own nutritional needs. Moreover, we found that while women's nutrition has been extensively studied as it affects pregnancy outcome, lactation, and infant growth and development, little attention has been paid to the nutrition of women beyond their childbearing roles. Studies on diet supplementation of pregnant and lactating women and the effects on pregnancy outcome of their diets and prepregnancy nutritional status abound. But little is known about women's lifelong diet, its effects on their short- and long-term health and well-being, the factors affecting this diet, and the ways policies can be developed to improve women's diet and nutritional status.

Our interests in this topic evolved at the same time that the Office of Nutrition, United States Agency for International Development (USAID), Department of State, was initiating its maternal and infant nutrition project. We discussed our ideas with Office of Nutrition Staff, who with other USAID health and nutrition officials decided to provide us with a grant to review women's nutritional status. Concurrently, interest in the role of maternal diet and nutrition as they affect fecundability, breast-feeding, pregnancy outcome, and ultimately, fertility, led the Carolina Population Center and its director, Dr. J. Richard Udry, to supplement funding for the review as the first step in a series of empirical studies we envision on this topic. At a final stage, we received additional support from the Nestlé's Coordinating Center for Nutrition in Washington, DC; this funding paid for editing and typing the final manuscript.

Many people have helped us in completing this review. The list of individuals who have provided us with materials, met with us, or sent us ideas and suggestions appears as Appendix A. We wish to thank especially Gayle Gibbons of the Infant and Maternal Nutrition Clearinghouse of the American Public Health Association and the Office of Nutrition of USAID for their assistance. In addition, we wish to thank Dr. Monica E. Yamamoto, who wrote the sections on the effect of women's diet and nutritional status on lactation and family planning programs. Dr. John Akin of our CPC research group has been of great assistance in the review and preparation of the manuscript. Helen Brown was most helpful during the final revision. Lynn Igoe edited the manuscript at various stages and prepared the index. Margaret Mauney served as proofreader.

Several persons have acted as primary consultants on the project. Foremost is Dr. Abraham Horwitz, director emeritus of the Pan American Health Organization (PAHO), Chairman of the National Academy of Science International Nutrition Committee, Chairman of the United Nations Coordinating Committee on Nutrition, and presently consultant at PAHO. He assisted in the design of the project, provided guidance in obtaining funds, and reviewed the manuscript. We also wish to thank Dr. Joseph C. Edozien, Chairman of the Department of Nutrition at the University of North Carolina at Chapel Hill; Dr. Sandra Huffman, nutritionist and assistant professor at the Johns Hopkins University Institute of Hygiene; and Dr. Janet Bauer, an anthropologist and then postdoctoral fellow at the Carolina Population Center for their consultation and suggestions on this document. Dr. Bauer developed the section on cultural determinants.

The views and interpretations in this document are those of the authors and should not be attributed to the Agency for International Development or to others who have provided assistance.

Barry M. Popkin

Chapter 1
Introduction

This report attempts to document the current state of nutrition research and practice concerning women during the reproductive years (generally ages 15 through 45) in developing countries, and to identify areas for future research and policy and program development.

Economic development strategies in low-income countries have frequently been criticized for ignoring women's economic roles and needs in income-generating activities, education, training, and technology transfer, instead directing women to training in child care and homemaking (Buvinić 1976). Furthermore, the perspective of research and programs in women's nutrition has generally been to examine women within the context of their childbearing role. Much nutrition research has focused on the consequences of women's diet and nutritional status during pregnancy and lactation because of their extreme importance for mortality and morbidity of both mother and child. Nutrition programs targeted at women generally provide diet supplements and/or nutrition education only during the reproductive phase, with infant health and development considered to be the key outcomes. Health programs similarly emphasize the provision of prenatal care and family planning.

While we in no way underestimate the importance of women's nutrition during pregnancy and lactation for the optimal health of mother and baby, we wish to establish a broader perspective for examining women's nutrition. Women not only have a unique biological role as childbearers, they also fulfill well-delineated social, economic, and cultural functions. The nutritional implications of the complex interactions between these biological and socioeconomic roles need to be examined not only during pregnancy and lactation, but also during the nonpregnant phases of the reproductive years.

1

We examine what is known about the nutrition of adult women in low-income countries. In Chapter 2 we review evidence of the significance of women's nutritional status and diet. What are the important functional consequences of women's nutrition that warrant consideration of women as a special group? We review research not only on the nutritional impacts on pregnancy outcome, fertility, and lactation, but also on productivity and morbidity.

In Chapter 3 we present evidence on what is known about women's nutritional status, diet, and pregnancy outcomes (birth weights) in low-income countries. We briefly review indicators useful for assessing nutritional status. In Chapter 4 we discuss various individual, household, and community factors considered determinants of women's food intake and nutritional needs. Chapter 5 is a brief summary of Chapters 2 through 4. Chapter 6 is a descriptive, analytical and evaluative discussion of nutrition and development programs which affect women's nutrition. We conclude with a summary of policy and program implications that arise from the review. Instead of setting out specific programs or policy options for any country or region, we summarize the various biologic and sociodemographic issues nutrition planners and policy makers should address when considering the nutritional needs of women.

Research findings on many topics covered in this review are scarce, and sample sizes frequently small and nonrepresentative. However, we feel that the data on the nutritional status, dietary patterns, and morbidity of women--and the determinants and consequences of these patterns--are adequate to warrant the broad perspective, inferences, and conclusions of this book.

Chapter 2
Significance: The Functional Consequences of Women's Nutritional Status

In this chapter we review current knowledge on the important consequences of a woman's nutritional status and diet during her reproductive years. Research in this area has focused predominantly on the nutritional impacts on pregnancy outcome, lactation, and fecundity/fertility. Most studies concentrate on the functional outcomes of moderate and severe malnutrition. Much less is known about the effects of mild or marginal malnutrition. Morbidity and productivity are two dimensions of women's health that malnutrition at varying levels of severity may affect. These issues have received much less attention for adult women, possibly because they have not been considered a high research priority and also because of the methodological difficulties associated with measuring what may often be subtle outcomes. We present information that highlights the need for further investigations of some of the significant outcomes of women's nutrition in terms of general health, childbearing, and nonchildbearing roles.

NUTRITION AND PREGNANCY OUTCOME

The impact of maternal nutritional status on pregnancy outcome and infant development has been the primary focus of research on maternal nutrition in low- and high-income countries. Two excellent and extensive reviews of the subject are Stein et al. (1975) and Susser (1981). Since we intend in this review to broaden the scope of research on women's nutritional status, we present only a brief review of the impact on pregnancy outcomes.

Birth weight and mortality (neonatal, perinatal, and infant)[1] are considered the most important commonly used indicators of reproductive success. Birth weight has been used to indicate infant health status and predict future health problems. Infants classified as having low birth weight (LBW--less than 2,500 grams), particularly those born preterm (gestational age less than 37 weeks), suffer higher neonatal and perinatal mortality rates and require more medical attention during the first year of life (Brimblecombe et al. 1968; Chase 1969). Studies in Guatemala indicate that infant mortality in babies weighing 2.5 kilograms or less at birth is nearly twice that of babies weighing more than that (Lechtig et al. 1975a).

Nutrition during pregnancy influences human fetal growth, although the mechanisms of this relationship have not been identified. Evidence of a relationship has been based largely on animal investigations, on studies assessing the impact of food supplementation during pregnancy (Lechtig et al. 1975b, c; Mora et al. 1979; Rush et al. 1980), and on epidemiological studies (Stein et al. 1978). Metcoff et al. (1979) note that mothers with no evidence of serious malnutrition can deliver fetally malnourished infants and conversely that poorly nourished women can deliver infants of normal birth weight. They suggest that pregnancy outcome may be more closely related to the mother's nutrient pattern or profile (nutrient imbalance) during pregnancy, than to excesses or deficiencies of specific nutrients.

A number of studies have examined the effects of prenatal nutritional supplementation on pregnancy outcomes. None has examined the differential effects of dietary supplementation on gestational age and birth weight.

A Guatemalan workshop (Lechtig et al. 1982) focused on the findings of seven studies which examined the relationship of supplementation and pregnancy outcome. In these studies, supplemental calorie and/or protein intake was consistently associated with increased birth weight among women at risk of producing low birth weight infants (Blackwell et al. 1973; Chávez 1978; Lechtig et al. 1982; Mora et al. 1979; Stein et al. 1978). In most of these studies supplementation improved birth weight by approximately 40 to 60 grams, with birth weight increments of up to 180 grams in supplemented Mexican women (Chavez 1978), and 400 grams in postfamine Dutch women (Stein et al. 1978). While the rise in birth weight associated with prenatal supplements seems modest, the degree of the rise may be modulated by other factors. In one study, prenatal diet supplementation of New York women appeared to protect somewhat against fetal growth retardation under the specific condition that mothers were heavy cigarette smokers (Rush et al. 1980). A study of Colombian women found maternal supplementation increased women's weights in both initial low and high calorie intake groups, but only improved birth weights for infants of women with high dietary intakes. These findings suggest a threshold exists which must be surmounted by effective supplementation before birth weights will increase (Christiansen et al. 1980). The Dutch famine study indicated that prenatal diet affects birth weight only when diet falls below a threshold level that approaches severe food deprivation (Stein et al. 1978).

Factors such as the quantity, type, and duration of supplementation; the timing of its introduction; and the severity of prepregnancy maternal undernutrition may account for the range of results in prenatal supplementation studies. The studies provide no conclusive evidence about the differential value of providing caloric or protein supplementation. In the Guatemalan study, birth weights were similar in protein- and calorie-supplemented villages (Lechtig et al. 1982). For New York women, a high protein supplement was associated with more prematurity than among women receiving either a balanced protein-calorie supplement, or no supplement (Rush et al. 1980).

The appropriate time to introduce a prenatal nutrition supplement also remains uncertain. Several studies indicate that supplementation during the last trimester of pregnancy can increase birth weight. Lechtig et al. (1982) conclude that total calories provided influences birth weight more than when they are introduced, but that supplementation begun earlier and sustained throughout gestation would be more likely to have additive effects. There are other indications that under extreme conditions of undernutrition, first trimester supplementation is most effective in lowering perinatal mortality rates (Stein et al. 1978).

Weight gain during pregnancy may influence both pregnancy outcome and postpartum maternal nutritional reserves. Some studies have found a strong correlation between weight gain and birth weight (Eastman and Jackson 1978; Hardy and Mellitta 1977; Naeye et al. 1973; Picone et al. 1982). Others have found statistically significant differences in the weight gain of supplemented and unsupplemented mothers which have not consistently been reflected in increments in mean birth weight (Christiansen et al. 1980; Rush et al. 1980). Metcoff et al. (1979) found a statistically significant but not strong association between total weight gain and birth weight. The weight gain of mothers in this study accounted for less than 5 percent of the variance in adjusted birth weight. A study in Kenya showed a low incidence of low birth weight (6.5 percent) despite average pregnancy weight gains of 6.5 kilograms for rural women and 7.9 kilograms for urban women (Jansen et al. 1980).

It has been difficult to establish a cause-and-effect relationship between diet during pregnancy and pregnancy outcome, since inadequate diets are also usually associated with other pregnancy risk factors such as poor living conditions, inadequate prenatal care, increased physical activity (Briend 1980), and exposure to disease. In addition, women at nutritional risk during pregnancy have generally had a poor nutritional history during the growth years. Maternal height is associated with birth weight (Drillien 1974; Fedrick and Adelstein 1978; Habicht et al. 1973; Keeping et al. 1979), but the association seems related to the correlation between height and prepregnancy weight, which is a strong determining factor (Bergner and Susser 1970; Kennedy et al.

1979; Pitkin 1979; Van den Berg 1977). Some studies in Guatemala indicate that maternal height and weight at conception may have a more significant effect on birth weight than caloric supplementation during pregnancy (Habicht et al. 1973). Studies also show that prepregnancy weight and weight gain during pregnancy can influence birth weight independently of each other (Eastman and Jackson 1968; Habicht et al. 1973). A low prepregnancy weight followed by a high pregnancy weight gain may result in a mean birth weight similar to a high prepregnancy weight followed by a low weight gain during pregnancy (Eastman and Jackson 1968).

While findings on the significance of nutrition for pregnancy outcome remain inconclusive, evidence suggests if preconception nutritional status is to be optimal for infant survival, efforts to improve it should begin in childhood. In addition, underweight women should be encouraged to increase their dietary intake during pregnancy as a means toward optimizing pregnancy outcome.

NUTRITION AND FECUNDITY/FERTILITY

The potential female reproductive years span menarche through menopause, a period of approximately 30 years. The upper limit to fertility (defined as actual reproductive performance or live births) is set by the woman's fecundity (reproductive capacity or ability to conceive) and then mediated by a number of fertility-inhibiting behavioral and biological factors. Nutritional status is one factor postulated to affect fertility. The links between nutrition and fertility have been the subject of several recent reviews (Bongaarts 1980; Menken et al. 1981; Underwood 1981; Zeitlin et al. 1983). Studies of chronically malnourished women have led to the hypothesis that malnutrition impairs fecundity (Frisch 1978a, b; Frisch and McArthur 1974). Other researchers conclude there is little support for a link between nutritional status and fertility in situations of chronic malnutrition (Bongaarts 1980; Menken et al. 1981). We will examine the evidence for a nutrition-fertility link in terms of the nutritional impacts on the biological components determining fertility: ages at menarche and menopause (the reproductive span); regularity of the components of birth intervals including length of the ovulatory period, lactational amenorrhea, and gestation; and the probability of intrauterine mortality.[2]

Age at Menarche

Great variations in age at menarche have been observed between females in developing countries and contemporary Western populations. The average age of menarche is about 13 years in modern Western societies (Tanner 1968), compared to an average menarcheal age in rural Bangladesh, for example, of 15.7 years (Chowdhury et al. 1977). There has been considerable debate about the relative importance of various biological, environmental, and socioeconomic factors thought to be determinants of menarche. Many investigators conclude that nutrition has a substantial effect on age at menarche.

Evidence indicates well-nourished females are likely to reach menarche earlier than poorly nourished women. Negative associations have been found between dietary intake and age at menarche (Frisch 1972) and height and/or weight and age at menarche (Chowdhury et al. 1977; Frisch and McArthur 1974; Hillman et al. 1970; Satyanarayana and Naidu 1979; Sogbanmu and Aregbesola 1979; Zacharias et al. 1976). These studies report differences of up to two years in mean age at menarche for females of high and low nutritional status. In addition, historical data indicate a decline in the age of menarche of about three years in European populations over the last century, which has been correlated with an increase in height and weight by age (Tanner 1968). In Bangladesh, where socioeconomic conditions have declined over the past decade in association with war, floods, and famine, Chowdhury et al. (1977) report an increase in the age at menarche which may be associated with the malnutrition accompanying these calamities. Poor socioeconomic conditions, closely linked to low nutritional status, have been consistently associated with higher ages at menarche in many countries (Burelle et al. 1961; Madhaven 1965).

While nutritional status appears to be correlated with onset of menarche, few investigators have attempted to explain the relationship. Frisch and McArthur (1974) propose that the onset and maintenance of regular menstrual function are each dependent on a minimum weight for height, representing critical fat storage. The mechanism proposed was that critical weight represents a particular metabolic rate which alters hypothalamic sensitivity to the gonadotrophins, resulting in increased gonadotrophin production and the initiation of menarche. A number of studies do not support the Frisch hypothesis. These investigators found neither the minimal variability of body weight and body fat at menarche Frisch proposes (Billewicz et al. 1976; Satyanarayana and Naidu 1979), nor that the majority of girls in each population achieve menarche at a weight that could be considered "critical" by either Frisch's designated level or that of the investigators (Billewicz et al. 1976; Satyanarayana and Naidu 1979; van 't Hof et al. 1977). Frisch's measure of relative fatness and statistical methodology have also been severely criticized (Trussell 1980). While changes in weight and body composition are clearly part of the maturation process, their possible role as a determinant of that process remains unclear.

For the undernourished female who begins menarche comparatively later, there is in many societies only a short interval between menarche and sexual exposure. Correspondingly, there is less time for optimum physiological and anatomical maturation before pregnancy. In general, adolescent girls do not complete linear growth until four years postmenarche (NRC 1970). Adolescents are likely to experience poor reproductive performance associated with the heavy physiological demands of pregnancy, undernutrition, recent or concurrent growth, and less than optimum physiologic maturation for reproduction (Wishik 1977). Age of menarche, and hence the beginning of potential childbearing, thus may have important nutritional implications for the young female, particularly in view of the early age at marriage and pregnancy characteristic of low-income countries. The overall effects on fertility of substantial changes in age at menarche following improvements in nutrition have been calculated to be small by some demographers (Menken and Bongaarts 1978). However, by simulating the effect on fertility of a two-year reduction in the age at menarche associated with improved nutritional status, Bongaarts (1980) calculates a concomitant increase of .25 births per woman, or a fertility increase of about 4 percent.

Age at Menopause

The complete cessation of menstruation at menopause signals the end of the reproductive years. Among Caucasian women, the mean age of menopause ranges from 49 to 51 years (Gray 1979). The limited number of studies in low-income countries indicates a wide variation in mean age of menopause, with a median age as low as 44 reported in Punjab, India (Wyon et al. 1966). Evidence on the determinants of age of menopause is inconclusive, probably because of methodological problems such as recall error in retrospective data and misreporting of age (Bongaarts 1980; McMahon and Worcester 1966). Studies have concentrated on the effect of various socioeconomic variables on menopause, with little mention of nutritional status as a potentially important determinant (Jaszmann et al. 1979; McKinlay et al. 1972). One study directly relating nutritional status to menopause reports that among malnourished New Guinean women, the median age at menopause was 43.6 years, while it was 47.3 years among better nourished women in a similar New Guinean population (Scragg 1973). A nutritional effect on age at menopause would have significance if it substantially altered parity among nonusers of contraceptives, and the additional pregnancies placed nutritional demands on an already marginally malnourished, high-parity woman. However, this effect is unlikely, since the latest age of childbearing seems substantially lower than the age of menopause for most populations.

Regularity of Ovulation

Frisch (1975) suggests undernutrition reduces reproductive efficiency causing a high frequency of irregular and anovulatory cycles. This hypothesis is based primarily on evidence of amenorrhea associated with the acute malnutrition of famine or the self-imposed starvation of anorexia nervosa (Antonov 1947; Frisch 1975; Keys et al. 1950). Evidence of the role of weight loss in amenorrhea remains inconclusive. Under conditions of starvation, significant numbers of women maintain regular menstruation (Keys et al. 1950). Of those who do become amenorrheic with weight loss, some studies report return of menses after restoration of normal weight (Crisp and Stonehill 1971;

Frisch 1975). Others report persistence of amenorrhea for long periods after ideal body weight has been achieved (Brasel 1978). Menstrual cycles may also cease without weight loss, associated with such factors as emotional stress (Rakoff 1968). Newton (1972) presents clinical evidence that malnutrition in women is associated with irregular menstrual cycles and a higher frequency of anovulatory cycles.

Frisch (1975) proposed a way that nutritional status may affect reproductive function. She suggests that a minimum level of stored, easily mobilized energy is necessary to maintain ovulation and menstrual cycles. A weight loss of 10 to 15 percent of body weight generally reduces stored energy to a level below this critical minimum, and will be associated with cessation of the menstrual cycle.

The difficulty of measuring regularity of ovulation limits investigation of the proportion of women who ovulate irregularly or the significance of nutrition in the process. It is also unknown whether the menstrual cycles of chronically malnourished women are affected similarly to those experiencing involuntary or voluntary starvation. Further evidence is therefore needed to substantiate a claim that chronic mild or moderate malnutrition affects regularity of ovulation, or that this has an appreciable effect on fecundity. There is also the bigger issue of involuntary sterility, estimated to affect about 5 percent of women worldwide, although there is little evidence to indicate an association with malnutrition (WHO 1975).

Lactational Amenorrhea

Particular attention has been focused on the ovulation-inhibiting effect of lactation as an important means of prolonging the birth interval. Reduction in the duration or frequency of breast-feeding speeds the return of ovulation following childbirth and thus increases fertility if contraception is not used (Delvoye et al. 1976, 1977; Howie et al. 1982; McCann et al. 1981). Nutritional status is one factor thought to explain the wide variation in the duration of postpartum amenorrhea reported among lactating women using no contraception. We discuss evidence for a direct effect of maternal nutritional status on postpartum amenorrhea. In addition, maternal nutritional status may importantly influence quantity and quality of breast milk and possibly the duration of lactation (see below). Since breast-feeding is the primary determinant of the length of postpartum amenorrhea (Delgado et al. 1979; Osteria 1978), maternal nutritional status may have an indirect effect through this latter pathway.

Several mechanisms have been proposed by which nutritional status may affect postpartum anovulation. The menstruation- and ovulatory-inhibiting effect of breast-feeding is believed to be caused by a hormonal reflex system initiated by the suckling stimulation (Tindal 1974; Tyson and Perez 1978). The hormone, prolactin, involved in milk production, and produced and secreted in response to the suckling stimulation, may interfere with gonadotrophic activity to prevent ovulation (Délvoye et al. 1978). Suckling frequency has been found in most cases to influence prolactin levels (Delvoye et al. 1977; Howie et al. 1982; Noel et al. 1974). Intensity of suckling may be the explanation (Tyson and Perez 1978). Aono et al. (1977) show that the intensity of the suckling stimulus is important for the amplitude of prolactin release. However, since this characteristic of suckling has not been consistently defined by researchers, further work is needed to verify these findings. The ovulation-suppressing effect of lactation may be reduced where infants are on a mixed feeding regime and suckling less frequently or less intensely.

Breast milk volume is adversely affected by poor diet and nutritional status (Edozien et al. 1979; Gopalan 1958; Paul et al. 1979a; Whichelow 1975, 1976; Whitehead et al. 1978). Lower breast milk volume may lead to more intense and prolonged suckling by the hungrier infant. Poorly nourished women may also have less access to supplementary food for their infants, and be more likely to breast-feed fully. Both situations may lead to higher frequency and intensity of suckling, stimulating prolactin release and more effective suppression of ovarian function.

Studies on the effects of maternal nutrition on suckling, per se, have been equivocal. Researchers in the Gambia found suckling frequency declined with an increase in maternal calorie intake (Whitehead 1982, as reported in Huffman 1982). However, in Bangladesh, the total amount of time spent suckling by infants 18- to 36-months old did not appear to vary with the mother's height--a proxy for nutritional status (Huffman et al. 1980a).

Results from the Gambia suggest dietary intakes may affect lactational amenorrhea by a direct physiological effect on prolactin levels (Lunn et al. 1980). The mean prolactin concentration profiles of three groups of lactating women of differing dietary intakes showed significantly different values. However, these results require careful interpretation since there was not careful measurement and statistical control of a crucial confounding factor--the child's suckling pattern--also, the definition of *infant feeding* was vague and the study did not consider breast-feeding time variations.

Frisch (1975) suggests that a critical percentage of body weight as fat is required to maintain regular ovulatory cycles, and that the energy demands of lactation prolong amenorrhea more in undernourished than in well-nourished mothers. Menstruation and ovulation would resume, therefore, only when sufficient weight and fat is regained postpartum. Evidence from Bangladesh does not support Frisch's theory, with a difference of only 1 to 3 percent between the mean weights of menstruating and amenorrheic women (Huffman et al. 1978b). In Guatemala women were losing weight throughout the postpartum period, regardless of the return of ovulation, indicating that resumption of ovulation was not triggered by weight gain (Bongaarts and Delgado 1979). In India, however, the weight of a lactating woman is inversely correlated with the length of postpartum amenorrhea when controlling for lactation duration (Prema 1981).

Several studies in low-income countries show an inverse association between indexes of maternal nutrition and length of lactational amenorrhea. In Guatemala, the difference in mean amenorrhea duration between high and low nutritional status groups defined on the basis of weight was 1.6 months, and defined on the bases of caloric intake was one month (Delgado et al. 1978). Among a Mexican population the length of postpartum amenorrhea was 6.5 months longer for unsupplemented women than for women receiving dietary supplements during pregnancy and lactation (Chávez et al. 1980). However, infants of supplemented mothers in the Mexican and Guatemalan studies also frequently received dietary supplements. Hence, decreased suckling by the infant, rather than the mother's improved nutritional status may have been related to the shorter duration of postpartum amenorrhea. More recent analysis in the continuing Guatemalan study indicates that improved maternal nutritional status during pregnancy and food supplements for infants during the first nine months of life are both independently and significantly associated with the length of postpartum amenorrhea (Delgado et al. 1979).

Data from Bangladesh indicate that poorer nutritional status had an effect in extending the length of postpartum amenorrhea. Chowdhury (1978) found a decline in the amenorrheic interval with increasing maternal weight, with a difference of 1.1 months of amenorrhea between women in high and low nutritional status groups. Another Bangladesh study contradicts Chowdhury's results. Huffman et al. (1978b) could not differentiate lactating women by weight-to-height measurements according to postpartum menstrual status. In an extension of this study, the median duration of postpartum amenorrhea for women in the lowest percentile of weight for height was only 2.4 months longer than for all women in the study (Huffman et al. 1980b). This constituted less than 10 percent of the average birth interval.

The difference of approximately one month in the length of postpartum amenorrhea in women of high and low nutritional status in Bangladesh and Guatemala suggests a small but important effect of nutritional status on postpartum anovulation. The potential impact on fertility of a change of this magnitude in the amenorrheic interval associated with improvement in nutritional status is calculated to be 3 percent (Bongaarts 1980).

Fetal Mortality

Fetal mortality has been estimated in the range of 15 to 20 percent of all pregnancies worldwide, although the rate in developing countries would be expected to be relatively higher (WHO 1975). From a prospective study in Hawaii which analyzed the probability of fetal loss by life table methods, French and Bierman (1962) estimated cumulative fetal loss among pregnancies over four weeks of gestation was 23.7 percent, with the highest losses at four to seven weeks.

Methodological problems limit the detection of fetal wastage and the assessment of the relative importance of various postulated etiological factors. Rates of intrauterine death are underreported, particularly in low-income countries (Potter et al. 1965; Retel-Laurentin and Benoit 1976).

A number of health, nutritional, genetic, and environmental factors are postulated to be possible causes of fetal mortality (NRC 1970; WHO 1970b). There is little evidence for a significant effect of nutrition on fetal survival. Under conditions of acute starvation in the Dutch and Bangladesh famines, there was no apparent increase in fetal deaths (Chowdhury et al. 1977; Stein et al. 1975). However, Antonov (1947) reported a doubling of fetal wastage in 1942 during the seige of Leningrad. Thomson (1959) suggests that women exposed to conditions in childhood which favor maximum skeletal growth and minimize pelvic abnormalities are less likely to be vulnerable to pregnancy wastage.

NUTRITION AND LACTATION

Maternal diet and nutritional status have been examined in relation to lactation performance, including milk quantity and quality and the duration of lactation.

Breast Milk Quantity

Maternal diet influences breast milk quantity to some extent. Whichelow (1975, 1976) reports on successful and unsuccessful lactation among well-nourished British women. Unsuccessful lactating mothers did not appreciably increase energy intakes during lactation as compared to their nonpregnant intakes, while successful ones did. Further, those on reducing diets noted an immediate reduction in milk supply. Gambian village women have seasonal reductions in milk yields, which coincide with decreased caloric intake and increased caloric expenditures during the rainy season (Whitehead et al. 1978). Supplementation studies focused on increasing protein and/or total caloric intakes report increases in milk yields of 15 to 25 percent (Edozien et al. 1979; Gopalan 1958). These findings need to be interpreted with caution in the cases of the Whichelow and Edozien studies because of very small sample sizes. The Gambian findings have also been questioned since important influences on milk yields, such as mean suckling frequencies, infant supplementation with other foods and/or milks, and maternal breast-feeding time allocations are not reported (Sandra L. Huffman, letter, 14 July 1981).

Studies of the effect of other indicators of maternal nutritional status on breast milk quantity have been few. Two Gambian studies provide interesting insights. Whitehead et al. (1978) found that among primaparous village mothers, milk yields increased through the infant's ninth month of age. Higher parity mothers, on the other hand, experienced their highest yields when their infants were three months old, with declines in milk yields thereafter. The researchers postulate that chronic malnutrition and nutritional depletion after repeated pregnancies may be a major factor in reducing the capacity to produce adequate milk yields. Another Gambian study (Paul et al. 1979a, b) reported that milk was significantly negatively correlated with changes in the mothers' skinfold thickness--gains in thickness were associated with lower milk yields. Paul et al. suggest there may be a competition between replenishment of maternal fat stores and the quantity of milk produced.

In summary it seems caloric intake may have an important influence on the quantity of milk produced, with reduced intakes rapidly affecting milk output and dietary supplementation increasing yields.

Some evidence indicates there may be a significant relationship between maternal nutritional status during and perhaps before pregnancy which can influence milk yields in the later stages of lactation. Additional work is needed to clarify this issue.

Breast Milk Quality

Several studies examine the effects of maternal diet and its supplementation on breast milk quality. Maternal dietary intakes of water-soluble vitamins (ascorbic acid, thiamine, riboflavin, pantothenic acid, and B12) as measured in both dietary intake analysis (Ingalls et al. 1938; Jathar et al. 1970; Rajalakshmi et al. 1974; Simpson and Chow 1956; Stuart and Connellan 1973) and supplementation studies (Deodhar and Ramakrishnan 1960; Deodhar et al. 1964) seem to influence the breast milk content of these vitamins. The influence of maternal dietary intakes of fat soluble vitamins is not clear although supplementation studies with vitamin A dosing (Kon and Mawson 1950) and introduction of vitamin A-fortified sugar (Arroyave et al. 1974) note a rise in vitamin A content of breast milk with prenatal and/or postnatal supplementation.

Some hypothesize that the total fat content of breast milk of poorly nourished women is diminished. Some published information on variations in total fat content of breast milk has uncovered differences due only to diurnal variation (higher fat content in the mornings) and stage of the suckling episode (higher fat content in the end or "hind milk"). Changes in fatty acid patterns are associated with differences in maternal dietary intakes (Youri et al. 1982). Mothers on high polyunsaturated fat diets show an increase in the polyunsaturated fat content of breast milk; mothers on calorie-restricted diets have a breast milk fatty acid pattern similar to maternal depot fat; and an increase in maternal dietary carbohydrate calories increases lauric and myristic fatty acids in breast milk (Insull et al. 1959). Clearer relationships have been found in Gambia between breast milk fat concentrates and maternal subcutaneous fat stores than with levels of maternal dietary energy intake (Prentice et al. 1982). The significance of these variations in the breast milk fatty acid pattern on infant nutrition and/or health remains to be clarified. Research is being conducted in the Gambia, Bangladesh, and Peru.

Total protein content of breast milk in study populations of well-nourished and malnourished mothers (Lindblad and Rahimtoola 1974) appears to be remarkably stable even under conditions of protein supplementation, although the proportion of specific amino acids may vary. Gopalan's early study (1958) on protein supplementation reports a similarity in overall protein intakes of exclusively breast-fed infants; however, milk quantity increased with the supplementation.

Little work has been done to examine the effect of maternal diet or nutritional status on mineral and trace elements in breast milk. Supplementation studies based on giving iron, copper, and fluoride did not find significant alterations in breast milk levels of these components (Filer 1977).

Studies of the relationship between maternal nutritional status and breast milk quality report impressive similarities between the breast milk composition (fat, lactose, nitrogen, vitamin A, and calcium) of undernourished women and well-nourished Swedish, Belgian, and Japanese women (Lindblad and Rahimtoola 1974).

In summary, some studies show little difference between breast milk quality of poorly and well-nourished mothers. However, maternal dietary intakes may significantly alter the nutrient content especially as the amino acid pattern, fatty acid, and water-soluble vitamin content of breast milk show. The question for further research is: To what extent would improvements in maternal diet be important to improved infant nutritional status? In other words, the studies which show increases in certain constituents of breast milk with supplementation do not clearly show whether such improvements actually improved infant health and/or nutrition.

Lactation Duration

Although there is currently much interest in the effect of maternal diet and nutritional status on lactation duration, little work has been done in this area (Delvoye et al. 1978). One study in Guatemala showed no effect of varying levels of supplementation on lactation duration, although prenatal and postpartum weight changes seemed associated with duration (Delgado et al. 1977). Chronically malnourished populations offer indirect evidence for the lack of impact of nutritional status on lactation duration; these women have extended durations of breast-feeding and the principal reason for weaning is a subsequent pregnancy (Huffman et al. 1980a).

MORTALITY AND MORBIDITY

Life expectancy in developed countries as a group is about 70 years, compared to 47 years in Africa, 49 in South Asia, and 61 in Latin America (UN 1979a). The low life expectancy in developing countries can largely be attributed to very high death rates among children (Golliday 1980). Women live longer than men in most parts of the world; see Table 1. In some countries women have higher death rates than men, particularly from ages 15 to 45. This reflects the increased risks of morbidity and mortality associated with childbearing (WHO 1980a).

Problems arise in analyzing data on the leading cause of death. In developing countries, many deaths are registered without identification of causes; multiple causes of death leads to misreporting; deaths may not be recorded; and data may not be sex disaggregated. In most developing countries complications of childbirth are among the five leading causes of death for women aged 15 to 44 (WHO 1980c), particularly postpartum hemorrhage, sepsis (infections), and hypertensive disorders of pregnancy (toxemia). Nutritional factors have been associated with all these factors. Antepartum and postpartum hemorrhages are more frequent in anemic women and are often more likely to be fatal for the anemic woman who cannot afford to lose blood (Fernandez 1971). Maternal mortality from puerperal sepsis was 34.4 percent in Latin American women with chronic anemia compared to an overall rate of 13 percent (Castelazao-Ayalia, 1971). We discuss the role of nutrition in toxemia later. Adequate nutrition, preventive and curative medical care could prevent most maternal deaths (Buchanan 1975).

Lack of a standard definition of *maternal mortality* and a scarcity of reliable data make intercountry comparisons of maternal mortality figures very difficult. As a brief comparison, a maternal mortality rate for the United States of 12.8 per 100,000 births (1975) compares to rates of 123 in Mexico, 126 in Chile, 249 in Iran, 370 in India, 570 in Bangladesh, and 700 in Afghanistan (Borazjani et al. 1978; Chen et al. 1974; Rao 1979; Taffel 1978; WHO 1980a).

Infectious and parasitic diseases, which appear in some countries to be a leading cause of death (Table 2), are associated with nutrition indirectly in terms of host susceptibility to infection. Other leading causes of death, including diabetes mellitus, hypertensive disease, and cardiovascular disease, are thought to have a nutritional component in their etiology.

Reliable information on disease patterns is unavailable on a countrywide basis for most nations. In addition, health data have often not been broken down according to sex, which makes it more difficult to determine women's health status. The coverage of services and facilities (from which most health statistics are collected) for women has been low, and priority has not been given to collecting information on female-specific conditions (WHO 1980a).

Nutritional anemia ranks among the four most prevalent serious nutritional problems in the world, together with protein-energy malnutrition, xerophthalmia, and endemic goiter (WHO 1972). *Anemia* is generally defined as a significant reduction (below a standard level) in hemoglobin concentration and/or red blood cells (hematocrit). Whereas protein-energy malnutrition and xerophthalmia have a higher prevalence among infants and children, anemia usually occurs most frequently among women of childbearing age. It occurs two to three times more frequently in nonpregnant women than in men, and up to 20 times more frequently in pregnant women (Buchanan 1975). Data on approximately 500 million women in developing countries indicate that about half the nonpregnant women and nearly two-thirds of the pregnant women have hemoglobin concentrations indicating anemia (WHO 1979). The overall proportion of women and pregnant women with below standard hemoglobins is highest in Oceania and Asia, followed by Africa and then Latin America (see Table 3). Extensive information on the anemia prevalence among women by country is available elsewhere (WHO 1979).

Anemia is important because of its diverse physiological and psychological sequelae, including lowered work capacity, lassitude, lowered resistance to infections, and increased complications of pregnancy and childbirth. With nutritional anemia the hemoglobin content of the blood is lower than normal because of a deficiency of one or more essential nutrients--usually iron, less frequently folate or vitamin B12. Nutritional anemia reflects an imbalance between the body's need for and absorption of the three nutrients. The balance can be disturbed by one or more factors which lead to a relative or absolute deficiency of the nutrient: (1) increased losses, (2) increased requirements, (3) decreased intake in the diet, (4) decreased absorption, and (5) decreased use. Some of the important specific components of these various factors include a generally low total food intake, as well as specific dietary deficiencies in iron, folate, or vitamin B12; loss of iron through menstrual bleeding, parasites, and diseases such as malaria and schistosomiasis; decreased absorption of iron due to other inhibitory substances in the diet, or a preponderance of less easily absorbed iron from vegetable sources; and the increased requirements for the three during pregnancy and lactation.

Nutritional deficiency diseases, other than anemias, have been greatly reduced in many developing countries through implementation of measures for their eradication. This applies, for example, to pellagra, beriberi, rickets, and scurvy for which available data suggest low prevalence (D.S. Miller 1979). A nutritional deficiency disease which still constitutes a public health concern in some regions of the world is goiter. A dietary deficiency of iodine has an etiological role in the development of goiter, which leads to thyroid disorders and cretinism. Kelly and Snedden (1960) report a 10 percent prevalence of goiter in developing countries. More recent sex-disaggregated data on goiter prevalence could not be found.

Infectious diseases, particularly intestinal parasitic and diarrheal diseases, airborne diseases, and vector-borne diseases, are the major causes of morbidity in low-income countries. The prevalence of infectious diseases is usually grossly underestimated because of the many factors leading to underreporting of disease in developing countries. The data are also usually not sex-disaggregated. Assessing the prevalence of infectious disease among women is therefore very difficult. Recent global prevalence estimates of two major infectious diseases were 180-200 million for schistosomiasis and 150 million clinical cases of malaria (WHO 1980d). Nutritional status increases the susceptibility to and the severity of infection as well as the functional effects of the disease (Latham 1975; Rosenberg et al. 1976; Scrimshaw et al. 1966). Multinutrient deficiencies, as well as deficiencies, imbalances, or excesses of single nutrients can lead to immune system dysfunction. The major nutrients that in deficiency states have been associated with immunological changes in humans are iron, folic acid, and zinc, and also excesses of essential fatty acids (Beisel et al. 1981). Imparied immunocompetence increases susceptibility to respiratory, dermal, intestinal, or systemic infections and contributes to high mortality.

There has been a good deal of controversy about the impact of nutritional factors on the development of complications of pregnancy, particularly toxemia. *Toxemia*, defined as hypertension with proteinuria and/or edema (NRC 1970), has been associated with important alterations in the growth and development of fetus and placenta (Alvarez et al. 1972; Hendricks and Brenner 1971). Studies have associated toxemia with undernutrition at conception and poor pregnancy weight gain (Tompkins et al. 1955), excessive pregnancy weight gain, and abnormal weight gain patterns (NRC 1970). Some feel there is no scientific evidence linking deficiency or excess of any nutrient and pregnancy toxemia (Davies 1971). Improved prenatal nutrition by food supplementation among Guatemalan women showed a positive nutritional effect on only one aspect of toxemia--a decrease in diastolic blood pressure--with no effect on systolic blood pressure and proteinuria (Lechtig et al. 1978b).

Chronic Diseases

Death rates from chronic diseases are far behind those for infectious and parasitic diseases in most developing countries (Table 2). Because many degenerative diseases are chronic for a long period before becoming fatal, death rates highly underestimate the disease prevalences. Although these conditions have classically been considered "diseases of affluence," with the increased Westernization of life styles and a decrease in early deaths from other causes in developing countries, they appear to be on the increase. The role of diet in the development of many chronic, degenerative diseases is fairly well accepted in industrialized countries, although theories on the specific dietary factors involved and the exact mechanisms are still controversial. Etiologies of chronic diseases have not been as extensively studied in developing countries, so it is not clear whether the same causative factors apply. The following discussion is based primarily on results of studies in industrialized countries, with information from developing countries when available.

Hypertension. Hypertension in and of itself can lead to death but it is most important in industrialized countries as a risk factor for cardiovascular disease and renal failure. Dietary factors implicated in the etiology of essential hypertension include obesity and salt consumption. Some of the earlier information on the relationship between salt consumption and blood pressure was from population studies comparing the low incidence of hypertension among many traditional nonsalt-consuming societies with that of the U.S. and other industrialized countries (Dahl 1972).

Rates of high blood pressure are not insignificant in developing countries, especially in populations which have experienced urbanization and Westernization. In rural Jamaica, Miall et al. (1962) found that, depending on age, 12.9 to 55.6 percent of females showed pressures greater than 160/95 compared with a range of 10.9 to 35.2 percent of males. A similar high incidence was found among blacks in South Africa (Seftel 1978), whose mean blood pressure at every age was greater than that of London whites. See Table 4.

Mean blood pressure and rates of hypertension generally increase with age except in certain populations which have retained their traditional life styles. In these populations, mean blood pressures show no change with age (Page et al. 1974; Sever et al. 1980; Shaper 1972). Women appear to have higher blood pressures and rates of hypertension than men, possibly related to more obesity among women (Page et al. 1974; Seftel 1978; Sever et al. 1980) or to childbearing (Matsuo 1967). Some studies implicate salt intake (Page et al. 1974; Prior and Evans 1969) but no information is available on the relative intake of males and females.

Diabetes mellitus. Regarding the role of diet in the development of adult-onset diabetes, the current consensus is that obesity is a major risk factor. The etiology of the disease seems related to an overall excessive intake of calories rather than to any specific source of calories (sugar, carbohydrate, fat, protein). With weight in excess of 120 percent of the ideal weight for height, Westerners experience a doubling of the risk of developing diabetes (Bierman 1979).

The prevalence of adult-onset diabetes and its relationship to various environmental factors have been studied in a few developing countries (Table 5). Rates across and within countries vary considerably, and are often significant, especially in the recently Westernized Pacific islands. Urban groups (Martin et al. 1980) and high income groups (West and Kalbfleisch 1970) appear to have higher prevalence rates. The relationship with age seems to be bell-shaped, with a peak between ages 30 and 50. Declines after age 50 may reflect the earlier deaths among those with the disease. Obesity was related to higher prevalence in almost every study except in India (Rao et al. 1972) where the condition still existed in significant numbers amid a generally malnourished population. West and Kalbfleisch (1971) calculated a correlation coefficient of 0.89 between mean diabetes rates and percentage of population in excess of ideal weights for heights in several countries. Zimmet (1979) suggests that obesity may affect the timing of the appearance of the disease rather than whether an individual ever develops diabetes. Studying the relationship between diabetes and obesity is complicated by the tendency for weight to decrease in the disease's latter stages.

As with hypertension, women often have higher rates of diabetes than men. This may be related to higher rates of obesity (Florey et al. 1972; West and Kalbfleisch 1966). While parity may play a role in women's higher diabetes rates (West and Kalbfleisch 1966), the relationship disappears when age and weight for height are controlled (Florey et al. 1972).

Coronary heart disease (CHD). The role of diet in the etiology of CHD is still controversial. Obesity may be related to the risk of CHD primarily through its impact on other risk factors such as blood pressure and diabetes, but its independent association with CHD is unknown (Van Itallie 1979). It is fairly well accepted that higher plasma cholesterol levels are associated with increased risk of CHD. However, what role dietary intake plays in the determination of plasma cholesterol levels is not clear. While population studies have shown a relationship between mean intakes of saturated fats and plasma cholesterol levels, as well as with CHD rates, studies on individuals have generally failed to document such a relationship (McGill 1979).

Data on the prevalence of CHD in developing countries are scarce. Screening for the presence of CHD in living individuals is much more complicated than for other chronic diseases such as hypertension or diabetes. Therefore, studies usually report either death rates, or the prevalence of risk factors such as plasma cholesterol levels, obesity, or blood pressure. Soukupová and Průšová (1970) present mortality data from 33 countries on deaths due to ischemic heart disease (IHD); they include several developing countries (Table 6). The mortality rates for men were greater than for women. The study compared mortality rates to dietary data and obtained high correlations between IHD rates and mean intakes of calories, sugars, fats, and protein. In the Solomon Islands, Page et al. (1974) found very little evidence of electrocardiographic abnormalities normally associated with CHD. Heart disease (which includes all forms of diseases of the heart, not just coronary heart disease) is the number one cause of death in nine of ten countries in the English-speaking Caribbean (Sinha 1980); sex-disaggregated data are not presented. Seftel (1978) reports on low death rates due to CHD among blacks in Johannesburg, South Africa, and relates this situation to a variety of risk factors, including plasma cholesterol levels, high blood pressure rates, cigarette smoking, and alcohol consumption. Again, data were not available by sex.

The role of dietary factors in the etiology of CHD is confused by results from several studies of nonindustrialized populations. A high incidence of CHD in Ceylon is associated with a low fat diet and a relatively low plasma cholesterol level (Shaper 1972). Although the fat intake is low (55 grams per day compared with a United Kingdom average of 155 grams per day), most of the fat is coconut oil, high in saturated fats. Another example concerns nomadic tribes of East Africa who consume a high fat diet of milk, meat, and blood, yet have a low incidence of CHD (Shaper 1972; Taylor and Ho 1971). Possibly their high cholesterol intake suppresses endogenous production so that plasma levels are not significantly high. In neither of these cases were the sexes studied separately.

NUTRITION AND PRODUCTIVITY

Low labor productivity is frequently found in conjunction with undernutrition and low incomes. The critical dimensions of productivity that appear to be affected by nutrition include labor time, intensity of work, and the productive value of the work activities selected (Popkin 1978). Most nutrition and productivity studies have been conducted on males in salaried or piece-rate, highly labor-intensive, structured occupations. Whether the results can be generalized to female populations who frequently work under conditions with different organizational, technological, and motivational dimensions than males, is not known.

In a working lifetime, or over shorter periods of time, nutritional status may limit total work effort. Poor nutrition can decrease a person's working time by placing a ceiling on prolonged physical effort (Oshima 1967). In addition, poor nutritional status may decrease work time through its effect on increasing the incidence and severity of morbidity, and hence absenteeism. Several studies have shown that improved hemoglobin levels associated with iron supplementation were correlated with significant increases in the average time worked, and a decrease in days of work missed (Basta and Churchill 1974; Popkin 1978).

The productivity or intensity of work per unit of time increases as nutritional status improves. Some studies examining work output under wartime starvation conditions, or in controlled caloric supplementation trials, report that energy intake significantly influences work intensity and capacity (Keys et al. 1950; Kraut and Muller 1946; Viteri 1976). Other studies have not found a relationship between productivity and caloric consumption (Belavady 1966; Satyanarayana et al. 1972). The inconsistencies of the results perhaps reflect the methodological difficulties associated with this area of research (Popkin 1978). In four World Bank studies in Indonesia, India, and Kenya, two sets of results showed a correlation between work output and caloric status, while all four showed a correlation between hemoglobin levels and work output or endurance (Basta and Churchill 1974; Karyadi and Basta 1973; Latham and Brooks 1977). Caloric status correlated with work output only in those areas where no significant anemia was present.

Among anemic female tea pickers in Sri Lanka, Gardner et al. (1977) found a significant inverse relationship between hemoglobin levels and various treadmill tests of physiological capacity. The Sri Lanka studies are unique in that they included both studies of the association between anemia and women's work performance and the effect of iron supplementation on the quantity of tea these women picked (Edgerton et al. 1979; Gardner et al. 1977). After one month, significantly more tea was picked when hemoglobin concentration was increased by iron supplementation. Edgerton et al. found the degree of improvement was greater in more anemic subjects (those with concentrations of 6.0-9.0 mg/dl).

In a research review, Beenstock (1978) concludes that iron deficiency anemia may be a more important nutritional determinant of labor productivity than energy intake. Nutritional anemia affects work intensity by decreasing the blood's oxygen transporting capacity. Improved nutritional status may have important effects beyond labor productivity. Viteri (1971) showed that supplemented Guatemalan peasants spent more leisure as well as market time in physically active tasks than an unsupplemented group. Those with limited energy reserves rested more and when not resting, engaged in much less active leisure activities. The percentage fully active was 67 for those supplemented and 5 for the unsupplemented peasants.

Nutritional status may also affect selection of work activities. If higher paying jobs are more physically or mentally demanding, well-nourished workers would be expected to select them (Baldwin and Weisbrod 1974). Individuals may adapt to low energy intakes by choosing those activities that will be minimally demanding on their energy stores.

Studies focus almost entirely on the nutrition/productivity relationships in males, and their economic implications. However, the issue is of particular significance to females for several reasons.

Females have higher incidences of iron deficiency anemia, which appears to be one of the most important nutritional determinants of labor productivity. During pregnancy and lactation, when women have particularly high nutritional needs, work time and productivity do not alter significantly. A review of studies in 202 traditional societies finds the most common single pattern of work activity during pregnancy was to continue full duties until the onset of labor, and return to full work within two weeks postpartum (Jimenez and Newton 1979). Women frequently contribute work time and energy to both market and home production activities. These dual roles are usually examined from the viewpoint of time allocation. Few studies have examined how changes in women's nutrition may affect qualitative dimensions of their home production, such as in child care and food production. Supplementation of mothers improves mother-child interaction, supposedly by providing them with greater energy and increasing their potential capacity for physical effort and ultimately their active time for interacting with the child, in turn an important factor in child development (Chávez and Martínez 1975). There are perhaps other such outcomes in the nutrition-productivity relationship beyond work time and intensity that need to be examined.

Chapter 3
Patterns: Variations in
Women's Nutritional Status

We have discussed some of the major consequences of poor nutrition among women. Here we review what is known about nutritional status of women in developing countries by looking at worldwide patterns of indicators of women's nutritional status. We will consider dietary and anthropometric measures of nutritional health, and also review patterns in pregnancy outcomes which may be related to maternal nutritional status. The prevalence rates for certain diet-related diseases are also indicators of nutritional health, but these have been more fully discussed in the section on mortality and morbidity, in Chapter 2.

First, we briefly summarize techniques for assessing nutritional status in field situations in developing countries. Much of this information is useful for determining male nutritional status as well as female. While standards of reference for indicators are usually age- and sex-specific, there are no assessment methodologies, except for indicators pertaining to pregnancy, applicable only to women.

In defining the nutritional status of individuals, four basic methods are used: anthropometric, clinical, biochemical, and dietary studies. We evaluate these methods in Table 7. Each method is best used in combination with one or more of the others since one is not very precise or reliable when used alone. Assessment findings suggesting a nutritional abnormality should be considered a clue rather than a diagnosis.

See Table 8 for the most commonly used indicators in the field level assessment of nutritional status, with a brief description of their uses, advantages, and limitations.

PATTERNS

Nutritional Status

Comprehensive data on the nutritional status of women in developing countries are severely lacking. What information does exist is based primarily on very small samples and is restricted to data on pregnant and lactating women. National nutrition surveys, such as those conducted by the U.S. Agency for International Development and the Centers for Disease Control, have collected data mainly on the nutritional status of children. A few exceptional surveys of large regions (e.g., Kusin et al. 1979, 1980) have included detailed assessment of women's dietary, anthropometrical, and biochemical data. The problems inherent in the assessment methods and the lack of use of appropriate statistical techniques in many of the studies reviewed indicates the need for caution in examining the figures presented.

A quick glance at the accompanying tables indicates the wide variety in nutritional status among people in developing countries. While women (and men) in many populations studied have generally deficient diets, some traditional groups, such as the Tarahumara Indians of Mexico, have quite satisfactory diets, while many newly Westernized groups, such as the Polynesians, suffer from the problems of dietary excesses. Therefore, making broad generalizations is next to impossible. In the remainder of this section we discuss some of the common findings, although the results are clearly not true for all countries studied.

Dietary intake. See Table 9 as a reference for WHO dietary recommendations. Readers will want to keep these recommendations in mind in considering the summary of information from studies on women's nutritional status in developing countries (Table 10).

Caloric intake is often low among women, although a few populations show adequate intakes (Mexico, Tarahumaras, Korea) or excessive (Micronesia) ones. Deficiencies in caloric intake are common, regardless of physiologic status. In one study (Pasricha 1958) pregnant Indian women consumed less than nonpregnant women. In other countries they frequently consume more, but their diets are still deficient in calories. Lactating women generally consume more than their nonpregnant counterparts, but still not enough to meet the daily recommendations. Where intakes are reported by income, low-income women appear to consume less than their middle- and high-income counterparts. Not only do women consistently eat less than men, in a number of studies (Bleiburg et al. 1980; Desai et al. 1980; Florencio and Aligaen 1980), they consume, on the average, a smaller percentage of their recommended daily intake.

Protein intakes appear to be more adequate in most countries than caloric intakes. However, the reported figures do not consider that, when calories are deficient, protein will be used for energy. Another issue not usually reported in dietary intake data is the quality of protein consumed. That women often consume lower quality, vegetable protein while men receive the larger share of whatever animal protein is available is most strikingly apparent in data from the Upper Volta, where women consumed 0.8 grams of animal protein compared with men's consumption of 10.3 grams daily (significantly different at P> 0.01). On the basis of quantity alone, women often consumed a smaller percentage of their protein requirement than did men.

The adequacy of vitamin intakes varies greatly by culture. Thiamin appears to be a problem only in a few countries (Philippines, India--low-income lactating women, Brazil and Egypt). Riboflavin intakes are inadequate in almost every country reviewed, while niacin intakes are generally adequate. The adequacy of vitamin A intakes varies considerably, while most women (except those in Singapore, Iran, and the Tarahumara Indians) are deficient in their vitamin C intakes. Calcium and iron are the two minerals most commonly studied and in a majority of the countries reviewed, women are seriously deficient in their intakes of both.

Anthropometric data. Studies on the anthropometric measurements of women in developing countries are even fewer than dietary studies. See Table 11. Although women in some countries have weights far below the WHO reference weight (55 kilograms), for the most part, women's weights appear to be more adequate than their dietary intakes would seem to indicate. Two studies show low weight for height is less common among women than men (Brazil, Upper Volta). Curiously, in both studies, women consumed a smaller percentage of their recommended intakes than did men. The cause of this discrepancy may lie in the differences in the level and efficiency of energy expenditures between men and women. Whether this pattern holds true for other countries is not known. However, it does point out the fallacy of evaluating nutritional status on the basis of dietary intake measures alone.

The amount and pattern of weight gain during pregnancy seems to be a critical indication of pregnancy outcome. The average pregnant woman in Europe and the United States gains 10 to 12 kilograms. Several studies in low-income countries report average pregnancy weight gains of only two to seven kilograms (Hauck 1963; Thomson et al. 1966; Venkatachalam et al. 1970). See Table 11.

Biochemical data. Because of the sophisticated techniques necessary for their determination, biochemical indexes of nutritional status have generally not been measured in developing countries. What studies have been carried out have focused mainly on determining the prevalence, severity, and causes of anemia (discussed previously). In a study of migrant farm workers in Brazil, Desai et al. (1980) found 25 percent of the women had plasma carotene levels below that considered acceptable while 25 percent also had less than acceptable plasma vitamin A levels. Dietary intake studies among these same women revealed that the mean intake of vitamin A was only 23 percent of the recommended level. No information is given on the range of vitamin A intakes so it is impossible to determine what percentage of the women had intakes below the recommendation, but with such a low mean it is likely that the percentage with deficient intakes was higher than the 25 percent with low plasma levels. Again, this discrepancy is an illustration of the problems encountered in using dietary information alone to assess nutritional status.

Kusin et al. (1980) studied serum vitamin A and iron status (hemoglobin and hematocrit levels) of 1,229 nonpregnant women, 825 lactating women, and 151 pregnant women. The differences between pregnant and nonpregnant women were significant (P> 0.01) for all indexes. In the sample 13 percent of the nonpregnant, 7 percent of the lactating, and 23 percent of the pregnant women had serum vitamin A values lower than the very deficient level of 10 mg/100 ml and 45, 34, and 43 percent respectively, had serum values in the low 10-19 mg/100 ml category. The pregnant women had significantly lower hemoglobin levels (a mean of 11.2 vs. 12.6 and 12.5 for the other two groups). Twenty percent of the pregnant group had hemoglobin values below 10 whereas only 10 percent of the other two groups were in this low value category.

Pregnancy Outcome: Low Birth Weight

Low birth weight (LBW) is often considered a proxy measure of poor maternal nutritional status, although, as we pointed out earlier, birth weight is affected by a number of variables, of which maternal nutritional status is but one. However, birth weight and maternal nutritional status (both before and during pregnancy) are undoubtedly related. Therefore, the prevalence of LBW infants will be reviewed here as a suggestive indicator of maternal nutritional health.

Information on rates of LBW in developing countries is scarce (WHO 1980b). Most developing countries lack the sophisticated systems for registration of vital events that developed countries have. What data exist are usually taken from special surveys or hospital records rather than routine vital statistics collections. The surveys are often of births in hospitals to urban mothers who have had some prenatal care. These births are rarely representative of all births in any developing country, where a majority of the population is usually rural, and births usually occur at home without any professional prenatal care (Akin et al. 1982). Thus, the reported statistics are likely to underestimate the prevalence of LBW infants among the entire population.

A second problem with birth weight statistics is the question of accuracy. This includes both the accuracy of equipment used and of personnel using it. A third problem is that birth weight data is rarely related to gestational age. Low birth weight among fully matured infants (small for date) may be caused by different factors than among preterm infants.

Most of the information on low birth weight in developing countries comes from two reviews of the literature on the prevalence of LBW throughout the world (Boldman and Reed 1977; WHO 1980b). See Table 12. Since the WHO data cover numerous smaller samples for most countries in the world, we report only selected more recent data for most nations. It is impossible to develop time trend information without a close analysis of the sampling frame definitions and measurement techniques used in these surveys. In general about 17 to 19 percent of all infants in low-income countries can be categorized as LBW. Asia has the highest percentage (20), followed by Africa (15) and Latin America (11). Clearly LBW is a common problem in low-income countries and may reflect widespread malnutrition among women, including poor prepregnancy nutritional status, inadequate dietary intake, and low weight gain during pregnancy.

SUMMARY

Information is scarce on the overall nutritional status of women in developing countries or on specific nutrition-related problems. Dietary surveys are the most prevalent form of assessment and have uncovered rather serious dietary deficiencies, although most have been conducted on very small samples of primarily pregnant or lactating women. Most of these dietary inadequacies are not related to more definitive anthropometric and biochemical indexes, so it is difficult to draw conclusions about women's overall nutritional status. The prevalence of low birth weight infants and certain diet-related diseases can be viewed as functional indicators of nutritional health (although both LBW and the diseases mentioned are multifaceted in causation). LBW rates are certainly alarming in developing countries, and the prevalences among women of many nutrition-related problems, especially anemias, maternal mortality, and infectious diseases, is higher than in developed countries and often higher than among men in developing countries.

Without more complete data, it is not reasonable, at this point, to draw firm conclusions about women's nutritional status from traditional biologic indicators. One must also investigate the extent to which women are subject to socioeconomic conditions associated with poor nutrition. Together with the biologic indicators, these socioeconomic indicators give a clearer picture of the level of nutritional risk women experience in developing countries. We discuss many of the factors which play a role in determining women's nutritional status in Chapter 4.

Chapter 4
Determinants of Women's Nutritional Status

In our view, a number of factors (see Figure 1) combine to affect the dietary needs and intakes of adult women. The relative importance of these factors varies significantly between and within different countries. Anthropological, economic, and sociological studies on women have rarely considered women's nutritional status to be a unique area of investigation. Women's status involves a configuration of multiple roles and positions in different domains (Oppong 1980), and nutrition may provide an example of the way role and status are differentiated by gender at the household and community levels. Dietary needs and intake are determined by biological factors, such as life cycle variations in physiology and socioeconomic factors which include income and resources, time allocation, labor and food markets, government services, household infrastructure, cultural factors, knowledge and training, and environmental variations such as seasonal cycles and changes in residence. Together these factors have an impact on overall household dietary needs and the quantity and quality of food allocated to individuals within the household.

There is a vast body of recent literature directed toward understanding the status and position of women with respect to social behavior and autonomy. This literature suggests that while sexual inequality is universal, with women's status rarely being equal to that of men's (Giele and Smock 1976; Rosaldo and Lamphere 1974), the relative equality of women and men in different spheres is likely to change at different rates through time. We discuss women's differential access to education, work, income, assets, and health care in the following sections, particularly as these variables interact with biological factors to determine women's nutritional needs. Research indicates that the status of women is the result of a complex interplay of social, economic, and biological characteristics (Parker and Parker 1979). The complexities involved in the relationships between women's social position and food patterns has yet to be examined empirically. Whether women's roles and statuses affect their diet through control of and access to resources, through intrafamilial distribution and culturally specific preferences in the handling of food, or by other mechanisms, needs to be examined more fully. The cumulative outcome of life cycle variations in female nutritional needs and intakes also needs to be studied more systematically. Sex-related differences in nutritional and health status begin in childhood in some countries (Chen et al. 1981; Levinson 1974; Solon et al. 1978). Early anthropological studies like that of Richards (1948) have chronicled nutritional intake and the factors associated with it during various stages of development, without systematically analyzing the physiological implication of these variations. In this chapter we analyze the economic, sociocultural, ecological, and physiological factors thought to affect the nutritional intake and needs of adult women.

We do not attempt to give priority to the importance of the various determinants of nutritional status. Rather we try to make the nutrition planner aware of some of the conditions that may limit the effectiveness of particular nutrition programs in different regions or countries.

PHYSIOLOGICAL STATUS

Descriptions of the activities and roles of men and women in different countries suggest that their respective energy requirements, susceptibility to diseases, and vulnerability to nutrient deficiencies also vary.

Energy Requirements

Based on the energy costs of common activities in industrialized countries, a Food and Agriculture Organization/World Health Organization committee has estimated daily energy requirements (FAO 1971). For adult females, energy requirements by level of activity are 36 kcal/kg for light activity, 40 for moderate, and 47 for heavy activity; requirements for adult males are 42, 46, and 54 kcal/kg respectively. There appears to be little support for an explanation of these quite large sex differences being based on sex differences in body weight, fat-free mass, or basal metabolic rate (Durnin 1976). The reasons for the differences remain largely unclarified.

The major factors in the human energy system are energy intake, energy expenditure, and body weight. If energy expenditure increases, either energy intake should also increase or body weight decrease, if metabolic efficiency is to remain consistent. However, the system does not always conform to theoretical expectations, because change in any two of the factors does not necessarily produce a predictable change in the third (Hegsted 1974); this may be because of individual variation in the efficiency with which energy is used and other adaptive responses in the energy system.

Durnin (1976) argues that the sex differences in energy requirements may be associated with particular adaptations to environmental stresses. For example, women in some low-income countries may compensate for nutritional stresses by doing more tasks while seated. Greenfield and Clark (1974) found that activity among New Guinean women was reduced in pregnancy, particularly in the last three months, and during lactation, more so in the first six months. The women walked less, spent longer periods sitting, and worked shorter hours. In a comparative study of Chinese, Malay, and Indian women, the percentage increase of expenditure over resting metabolism in common activities was more in nonpregnant than in pregnant women, indicating that the latter performed tasks in a more relaxed and economical way (Banerjee at al. 1971). Despite the higher energy demands of the increased basal metabolic rate of pregnancy, an adaptive decrease in daily energy expenditure by some women may function to keep total energy requirements constant.

Sukhatme (1977) suggests there is an adaptive response of energy expenditure to intake. Adaptability of energy expenditure to a reduction in energy intake may function through the metabolic changes associated with reduced physical activity which reduce the amount of energy needed for maintenance energy needs. Body weight and activity may continue to decline over time until a new energy equilibrium is reached, albeit at a lower level of function (Longhurst and Payne 1979). The adaptive response of energy expenditure may be more or less immediate, or it may develop over a long period of exposure to low energy intakes, or in a community or ethnic group over generations.

In industrialized nations, activity-specific energy rates are well described (Durnin and Passmore 1967), and energy needs calculated for the "reference" male and female (NRC 1980). However, studies indicate that adult activity patterns differ significantly from those used in developing nutrition recommendations (Robinson et al. 1973). For populations of low-income countries, there is a lack of information on the energy rates of many activities, particularly those common to agrarian societies. In addition, there is a lack of representative data describing time allocation to various activities (Montgomery 1978). This information gap has particularly related to women's energy expenditure and time allocations.

In the few studies of women's energy expenditure in low-income countries, daily energy use seems in fairly close agreement with the FAO standards for moderately to very active women (40 to 47 kcal/kg). Rural women in highland New Guinea (Norgan et al. 1974) and lowland Peru (Montgomery 1978) have an average daily energy expenditure of 44 kcal/kg. McGuire (1979) measured an average daily expenditure of 40.7 kcal/kg by rural Guatemalan women. Neither the Peruvian nor Guatemalan studies found seasonal variations in women's energy expenditure, although seasonal differences in energy intake, expenditure, and in body weight have been reported in other geographical regions (Chen et al. 1979; Wilmsen 1978).

In the Upper Volta, female farmers had a mean energy cost of 42.2 kcal/kg in the dry season and 52.6 during the rainy season (Bleiberg et al. 1980). Male farmers in the same region were also moderately active during the dry season (40.2 kcal/kg expenditure) and exceptionally active during the wet season (57.7) (Brun et al. 1981). Considering the year-round energy expenditure of these Voltaic farmers, the women appear to be more overworked than males. Both sexes expend high levels of energy during the peak agricultural season, with males having a longer daily duration of hard physical work (7.3 hours a day vs. 3.7 for women). However, during the dry season men rest comparatively more (Brun et al. 1981). While body weight measured in this study did not reflect a significant seasonal negative energy balance, other studies of female Voltaic farmers showed an average weight loss of 2.2 kg and a reduction of 7 percent of the triceps skinfold thickness between seasons (Gentilini, M. and Froment, A., personal communication, reported in Bleiberg et al. 1980).

Montgomery and Johnson (1977) have emphasized the need for an ecological approach to the determination of energy requirements for population groups. Factors such as gender-typed task allocations, work settings, type of technology available to workers, and sex differences in quantity and performance of work have significant effects on energy expenditure (Montgomery 1978). The additional energy costs for women of pregnancy (300 kcal/day) and lactation (500 kcal/day) must also be considered. Energy requirements may be subject to cultural and individual variation depending on such factors as shifts in work activities associated with reproductive status, and the adaptive responses to an altered energy equation which have already been discussed.

Disease

Large segments of populations in developing countries are subject to diseases which have nutritional implications, often occurring concurrently with malnutrition. It is estimated, for example, that more than 150 million people per year are affected by malaria (WHO 1980d), and one billion by Ascaris (Peters and Gilles 1977). Since infectious diseases are the major concern in developing countries in terms of prevalence, research, and programming, we will not cover the nutritional needs associated with chronic diseases.

The impact of infectious diseases on nutritional needs has received a good deal of attention in low-income countries, but predominantly in relation to children rather than adults. Women deserve attention in this regard since the nutritional demands of illness may exacerbate already marginal nutritional status, or be compounded by the simultaneously high nutritional demands of pregnancy or lactation. Women may also be at greater risk of infectious disease since as mothers they are in contact with sick family members. In some countries, women who become ill are less likely to seek medical assistance than males (Golliday 1980). Unfortunately, few sex-specific disease incidence data exist to allow an analysis of the differential impact of disease on the nutritional status of adults.

The most widespread diseases in developing countries are the intestinal parasitic and infectious diarrheal diseases, the airborne diseases, and the vector-borne diseases (Golliday 1980). All infections, mild or severe, whether bacterial, viral, or parasitic, result in aberrations of nutritional balance (Scrimshaw et al. 1966). Infection increases loss of essential nutrients from the body, and generally interferes with food intake. Conversely, malnutrition, even when subclinical, affects one or more of the mechanisms of resistance to infection (Scrimshaw 1975). Scrimshaw et al. (1966) found that in 67 percent of 500 studies reviewed, nutritional deficiency apparently increased the severity of infection by viral, bacterial, or parasitic pathogens. In some cases, malnutrition decreases the virulence of the pathogen, and subsequent morbidity and mortality. Iron deficiency is reported to be antagonistic to E. histolytica, malaria, and other pathogens (Murry et al. 1978). The interactions of infection and nutritional status are reviewed in detail elsewhere (Rohde 1978; Rosenberg et al. 1976; Scrimshaw et al. 1966).

In addition to the acute changes in nutritional status produced by infectious disease, recent studies have focused on the problem of chronic subclinical infectious disease (Shiffman et al. 1978). It is believed to occur in a significant proportion of individuals living in tropical countries (Forsyth 1969; Greenham 1978; Jordan and Webbe 1969). One study found iron losses of up to 37.3 mg/day in patients with Schistosoma infection (Farid et al. 1968). There is considerable evidence that males are at greater risk or exposure to Schistosoma infection and to its urological complications (Bell et al. 1973; Forsyth 1969; Greenham 1978). Helminthic infections may aggravate the risks of anemia in women during the reproductive years when they are already susceptible to the iron losses associated with menstrual bleeding, pregnancy, and lactation.

Malaria is an infectious disease characterized clinically by fever, varying degrees of anemia, splenic enlargement, and other complications. In addition to the metabolic costs of fever, there are diverse host responses with nutritional consequences including anorexia, altered carbohydrate and fat use, catabolism of skeletal muscle, increased gluconeogenesis and nitrogen excretion, and an anabolic response with changes in the priorities for protein synthesis (Solomons and Keusch 1981). In endemic areas, such as tropical Africa, it is estimated that 80 to 90 percent of people are infected with malaria (Noguer 1980). Malaria is an important factor in the genesis of anemia during pregnancy (Gilles et al. 1969; Reinhardt 1978). Women may have decreased malaria immunity during pregnancy (Kortmann 1972). Malaria during pregnancy has been associated with increased fetal wastage and low birth weight (Kortmann 1972; Macgregor and Avery 1974). Controlled trial studies with antimalarial therapy have shown weight gain during pregnancy is lower in untreated mothers (Morley et al. 1964). In addition, transplacental passage of parasites can result in congenital malaria (Bradbury 1977; Woods et al. 1974). Possibly malaria suppresses lactation, although there is no evidence to date of this relationship (Noguer 1980).

While there is a good deal of evidence on the prevalence and consequences of parasitic disease among adults, less is known about these aspects of bacterial diseases. Bacterial diseases, such as some of the diarrheas and upper respiratory diseases, have been extensively studied among children, but our knowledge of their occurrence and nutritional significance among adults is limited.

In addition to the direct nutritional implications of disease, infections may alter the individual's ability to provide food for herself or her family. Some of the common infectious diseases in developing countries can lead to blindness, debility, low productivity, inability to care for oneself, and other sequelae that may indirectly affect nutritional status.

Life Cycle Variations in Nutrient Needs

Women's energy and nutrient requirements vary during different stages of the life cycle. Ethnographic data have described the changes in female activities and roles during puberty, menstruation, childbearing, and old age (Kendall 1968). During these periods women's physiological needs change and their susceptibility to disease (as suggested earlier) varies.

Pregnancy. Any consideration of female nutritional needs usually revolves around pregnant women, who form a nutritionally vulnerable group because of their increased nutritional needs. Pregnancy is accompanied by anatomical and physiological changes necessary to regulate maternal metabolism, promote fetal growth, and prepare the mother for labor, delivery, and lactation. Optimal function of these processes requires increased intake of energy and of all the nutrients hitherto examined by the National Research Council (1980).

There is general agreement that the energy cost of pregnancy per se is an additional 300 kcal per day, if the woman is to gain the 10 to 12 kg compatible with a favorable pregnancy outcome (NRC 1980). This represents an increase of approximately 15 percent over nonpregnant energy needs. This energy requirement does not take into account additional factors which may affect energy needs, such as physical activity, or growth needs of a pregnant teenage woman unrelated to gestation.

The protein requirement of pregnancy is estimated to be 30 grams per day, in addition to the basic daily allowance of 0.8 g per kg in the adult woman (NRC 1980). This protein allowance is for the mixed proteins of the United States diet, which may not be customary in many diets in developing countries which are usually based more on vegetable than animal protein. Increased amino acids are necessary for protein synthesis related to expanded maternal uterine, breast, and intercellular fluid, as well as for protein synthesis in the feto-placental compartment (Pitkin 1979). The metabolic interrelationship between energy and protein dictates that the daily energy intake should not fall below 36 kcal per kg if protein metabolism is to be maintained appropriately (Pitkin 1979).

There are additional pregnancy requirements for all vitamins and minerals, which increase approximately in proportion to the increase in energy needs. There is, however, controversy as to whether the requirements for certain nutrients, such as folate and iron, are increased to such an extent that it is difficult to meet them through increased dietary intake alone. The substantial iron and folacin needs of pregnancy are caused by increased erythropoiesis, in conjunction with expanded blood volume and maternal-fetal nutrient transfer.

Scientific knowledge of nutritional physiology during pregnancy has been gathered mostly from well-nourished women. Relatively little is known about the physiological modifications and adaptive limits of pregnancy that may occur in chronically malnourished women, or how well dietary recommendations can be applied to pregnant women with a history of marginal or severe malnutrition.

Earlier we discussed women's dietary patterns, showing that pregnant women rarely consumed the additional 300 kcal per day they required. Two rural Mexican studies show exceptions where pregnant low-income women consumed about 250 calories more than nonpregnant/nonlactating women (Martínez et al. 1977). The more usual case is rural East Java where inadequate diets of pregnant women were substantiated by low pregnancy weight gain and relative loss of weight in the last trimester (Kusin et al. 1979).

The nutritional requirements of pregnancy have received extensive coverage in the literature. Since the subject is only a small part of this review, the reader is referred to other sources for more comprehensive discussions (Hytten and Leitch 1971; Pitkin 1979; Thomson and Hytten 1978; Thomson et al. 1979; WHO 1979).

Lactation. The committee on Recommended Dietary Allowances (NRC 1980) recommends significant increases in protein and energy intake for the lactating woman, and more moderate increases in the intake of all other nutrients. An additional 500 calories in the daily diet during the first three months of lactation is advised, assuming the mother has gained adequate weight during pregnancy. In low-income countries, women frequently have suboptimal gestational weight gain. Additional energy needs should be based on the requirement of an 80-95 kcal energy intake to produce 100 ml of milk, considering a daily breast milk production of 850 ml to be adequate. Women in developing countries produce usually much less than 850 ml of milk. If lactation continues beyond three months, if more than one infant is nursed, or if maternal weight falls below ideal weight for height, then the daily extra energy allowance should be increased accordingly. A 20-gram increase in daily protein intake is advised for lactating women.

Most dietary studies in low-income countries have found lactating women have inadequate dietary intakes according to recommended levels; calorie deficiencies are generally more prevalent and more severe than protein deficiencies (see Table 10). In several studies where lactating women consumed half the recommended calorie level, deficiencies were often in the range of 1,000 kcal. Lactating women generally increased their calorie intakes only slightly over the intakes of their nonpregnant, nonlactating counterparts, whose diets were already deficient. Thus it is likely that lactation may have a detrimental effect on a woman's nutritional status.

Although dietary intakes of lactating women--especially calories--are routinely inadequate when compared with recommendations, the impact on anthropometric and biochemical indexes is not so dramatic. Delgado et al. (1981) found after 12 months of lactation, supplemented women in Guatemala had lost only .90 kilograms over their first trimester weight, even though their calorie intakes averaged 70 percent of the recommendations. In a thorough study in the Gambia, Paul et al. (1979b) found lactating women lost weight only during the rainy season, a time of heavy agricultural labor and food shortages, when even nonpregnant, nonlactating women lost weight. At other times of the year, lactating women either maintained or gained weight, even with low calorie intakes. Other adaptive factors may operate to modify the impact of inadequate dietary intake during lactation on maternal nutritional status.

Effects of Contraception on Nutritional Status

The effects of various kinds of contraceptives on nutritional status is of vital concern to women's health during the reproductive stages of life. Women who use IUDs or who have a number of spontaneous or induced abortions are subject to heavy blood losses. The likelihood of these women developing iron deficiency anemia is increased, particularly if they already suffer from marginally deficient iron status.

Hormonal contraceptives are widely used in the family planning programs of developing countries. A number of studies have evaluated the effect of oral contraceptives (OC) on the metabolism and function of various nutrients. Alteration in the metabolism of vitamins (B6, B12, A, C, riboflavin, and folacin) and of some minerals (iron, zinc, and copper) is widely reported (Ahmed et al. 1975; Briggs 1976; Massey and Davison 1979; Prasad et al. 1977; Theurer 1972). Although evidence is conflicting, particularly concerning folacin and zinc, generally OC use is associated with increased serum levels of vitamin A and iron (because of decreased menstrual blood loss) and decreased serum levels of vitamins B6, B12, C, and riboflavin (Vitalis 1980). Some of these changes may be of no clinical significance but others may be of some concern. In addition to the effects of OC on vitamin nutritives, contraceptive steroids have also been associated with impaired glucose tolerance, elevated triglyceride levels, and altered protein and amino acid metabolism (Spellacy 1974; Warren 1973; WHO 1973).

Existing information on the metabolic effects and clinical implications of hormonal contraceptives has been based largely on studies of well-nourished women in developed countries with access to health care (Belsey 1977). The applicability of the finding to low-income women with nutritional disorders, marginal nutritional status, and suffering from a variety of endemic diseases has not been established. In addition, the majority of observed metabolic effects have not been assessed in terms of their long-term health consequences. Disease characteristics, particularly from diseases producing secondary nutritional deficiencies, may have important interactive links with the nutritional status of oral contraceptive users in low-income countries. A study in Egypt suggested that hormonal contraception may have a deleterious effect on liver function in the presence of schistosomiasis (Sakr 1973). In contrast, OCs have been associated with an improved rate of recovery from tuberculosis when used with adequate antituberculosis therapy (Mehrotra et al. 1974).

A further effect of oral contraceptives which has received considerable attention is that of lactation suppression. A number of studies have shown that combined estrogen-progestogen OCs appear to decrease breast milk volume or to shorten the duration of lactation in some women (Barsivala and Virkar 1973; Miller and Hughes 1970; Osteria 1978). Other studies imply that placebos are as effective as estrogens for suppressing lactation in women who do not want to breast-feed and have no effect on the lactation of women who do (Borglin and Sandholm 1971) Current evidence suggests that oral contraception should not be initiated during the early postpartum period until breast-feeding has been well established.

INCOME AND ASSETS

Income is a major determinant of the quality and quantity of household diet. Several trends in dietary patterns have been observed in many countries as income levels increase: (1) a reduction in the proportion of income spent for food, but a rise in absolute expenditure; (2) a decreased amount of calories from carbohydrates and increasing amounts from animal or vegetable proteins; (3) increased purchases of processed and in some cases relatively less nutritious foods (Berg 1973; Levinson 1974). While there may be some negative nutritional effects associated with higher income, the overall effect of increased income on a population is one of larger quantities and higher quality of food, and hence improved nutritional status (Chernichovsky and Kielmann 1978; FAO 1976a; Levinson 1974). A study in Brazil indicates income may be more decisive in determining the total amount of food available to a family, rather than the nutritional quality of the diet (G.R. Jansen et al. 1977). The sensitivity of nutritional quality to income may vary by region or country, however, depending on the relative contribution of annual, cereal, root, and bean products to the diet.

Assets which can both determine (e.g., land, farm implements) and be determined by (housing, cooking utensils) family income can have an important impact on household health and nutritional status. Total household food intake would be expected to improve with the improved purchasing patterns, storage facilities, and cooking methods generally associated with certain household assets. Increasing income and assets allows a family to purchase food in bulk, which usually means lower prices per unit. A household with a refrigerator can store food longer and more safely, reducing wastage. Other food storage facilities are also important in controlling food wastage from climate and pests. Quantity and quality of cooking utensils (in terms of heat conduction, for example) have substantial time costs associated with food preparation which can affect dietary quantity, variety, and nutrient losses. While little work has been done on the net impact of home assets on time allocation, their effect may be significant. For example, Herrin (1979) has discussed the effect of electricity on household time allocation patterns. Fuel is an important asset in terms of its time and money costs and the direct impact its availability may have on food preparation. With fuel shortages, diets may undergo transitions towards products that take less cooking time. Women may also make more use of cold leftovers, raw foods, and drink unboiled water, which can carry health risks, particularly in the absence of refrigeration (Hoskins 1979).

Low-income families frequently have less adequate household resources such as housing, water supply, and sanitation which indirectly affect nutritional status. The impact of a poor environment on disease patterns and prevalence, and the interaction of disease and nutritional status are reviewed elsewhere (Briscoe 1978; Kawata 1978; Shiffman et al. 1978).

The association between income and assets and the total value of food available to the household is well established. The effect of the mother's income on total family income, and on her diet, is unclear. Increases in the mother's wage may not necessarily be reflected in increased total family income, since she may be working to compensate for her husband's loss of income, or she may be the sole economic supporter of her family (Engel 1980). In addition, some evidence indicates that income earned by the mother goes more directly to her children than does income earned by the father (Safilios-Rothschild 1980). Guyer (1980) showed that cash expenditures of rural Cameroon women were dominated by food and basic supplies, whereas their husbands contributed only one-third of these expenses. Moreover, these women contributed over 30 percent of home-produced foods, estimated to account for as much as 45 percent of total household income.

A woman's access to and autonomy in the use of her own income or the total household income and assets would be expected to be a major determinant of her diet. This influences her options to purchase and consume food both within and outside the household or to trade food items within a social or marketing network. Within some cultures, the woman's contribution to the household income is a direct measure of her economic value. Some writers argue that for women, economic power is the most important influence on their relative equality, and therefore on their freedom in decision making, life options, and control of resources, such as food (Blumberg 1976; Sacks 1970). One of the consequences of urbanization and rural-urban migration seems to be that women increasingly lose their economically productive roles within the household unit. Often they are not allowed to assume income-generating activities outside the home, as men are (Boserup 1970; Giele and Smock 1976). There is, however, little evidence to indicate the effects of this situation on women's food intake or on their control over food resources.

In some societies females are the last to receive food, probably because they are not seen as economically central (Horowitz 1980; Valenzuela 1978). As a woman's contribution to the household income increases, so does her economic value to the family unit. The relative amount of household food she receives may improve as a result (Katona-Apte 1977b). Food distribution within the family may relate primarily to the economic value of each person's time (Mirrlees 1975; Underwood 1981).

Income may indirectly affect personal dietary needs through the limited jobs, assets, and resources available to low-income women. Poor women, particularly in rural areas, are more likely to engage in strenuous physical labor, which increases their energy needs. They have fewer household assets such as piped water and gas or kerosene stoves which are time and energy sparing. They cannot afford labor-saving purchases such as partially or totally processed or prepared foods, or child-care substitutes. Energy expenditures and needs are thus closely intertwined with income, and with time allocation decisions, discussed below.

Finally, income changes may affect women through the way improvements in household economic status improve their status. This issue is addressed later under the context of the impact of development programs on women's nutrition. However, research shows that improvements in household economic status not only may not improve women's status, but it may be accompanied by a deterioration in their status relative to men (e.g., Acharya 1981).

TIME ALLOCATION AND WORK

In developing economies, where households have limited access to physical capital and modern technology, time is one of the few resources available. The way time is used offers clues to the causes and consequences of poverty, and has thus been the subject of increasing interest in development studies (Birdsall 1980). The study of time has also provided some insights on how women may affect household nutrition. A woman contributes to the household economy by either transforming her time into income by engaging in market labor activities, or by using time to produce welfare commodities for the household such as child care, breast-feeding, and food (Evenson and King-Quizon 1978; Jayme-Ho 1976). Household nutrition can be viewed as a combination of both income (which is related to food purchasing) and time (a determinant of food production, preparation, and feeding) (Popkin and Solon 1976). Household work in low-income countries is time intensive, such that even small differences between households in the ease with which tasks can be done (for example, collecting fuel or carrying water) have important effects on other aspects of household welfare such as food production (Sharman 1970).

The total daily time that a woman engages in various activities and the types of work she does affect nutritional requirements. Women in developing countries commonly work longer hours per day than men, and engage in energy-intensive work, such that the nutritional demands of their work and time may be significant. In addition, a woman's allocation of time between household and market production may function as an important determinant of the diet of a low-income household. Time allocated to market activities affects household income, which is associated with food quality and quantity. Time allocation to market and household activities also determines the time available for food production and preparation. What evidence links these dimensions of time with nutritional status?

The time women allocate to market and home production activities appears to be significantly greater than that contributed by other members of the household (DaVanzo and Lee 1983; Evenson et al. 1979; Mueller 1979). As a consequence, women also have less leisure time than men, which has implications for the woman's energy expenditure and needs. Taking into account work and rest patterns over several seasons, women in some cultures are more overworked than men (see the seasonal variations section).

Women in Bangladesh, the Philippines, Nepal, and Upper Volta typically work 10 to 12 hours a day in household and market production whereas men daily work several hours less (Acharya 1981; Evenson and King-Quizon 1978; Farouk and Ali 1975; Hart 1975; McSweeney and Freedman 1980). In the Philippines, Evenson and King-Quizon found women worked an average of six to eight hours per day in household work and approximately three hours in market work, compared to males who spend close to one hour in household work, and seven to eight in market labor. Evenson (1979) reviews a number of time studies indicating that men rarely do more than one hour per day of household work. Women, therefore, frequently carry an economic responsibility for the household, and additionally, a domestic burden which is in most cases unshared by men. In Nepal, adult women worked 10.81 hours per day while men worked 7.51 and female children (aged 10-14) worked 7.44 hours compared to 5.31 for boys this age (Acharya 1981). Women in Upper Volta and Botswana (Kassoudji and Mueller 1980) work 20 percent longer and have 20 percent less leisure time than men (McSweeney and Freedman 1980). In Upper Volta while everyone works long hours and expends high levels of energy during peak agricultural seasons, men rest comparatively more than women during the dry season (Brun et al. 1981). The Voltaic men slept 0.7 hours longer than women, and sat inactively almost two hours more than their spouses per day during the dry season. This study clearly shows the effects of women's work on time available for food preparation. During the peak work season, women spent approximately 1.5 hours less on food preparation than during the dry season, serving only one hot meal a day and eating more leftovers and cold foods (Bleiberg et al. 1980).

The type of work women do has an impact on their caloric needs, their income-generating potential, and time they have available for food production and other activities. Labor force statistics are rarely representative of women's work since they fail to tabulate (1) work that does not produce cash income, (2) seasonal work, (3) workers in the informal sector, and (4) women whose main occupation is "housekeeping" even if they work part-time in jobs that would be counted as employment (Bruton 1980). The reported participation of women aged 15 and over in the labor force of developing countries is 22.6 percent as compared to 52.5 percent for men (ILO 1978). When agricultural labor on family farms is included in labor statistics, much higher proportions of women work. Women constitute over half the world's agricultural labor (Mickelwait et al. 1976), and up to 70 percent in rural Africa (FAO 1976b). Less than 20 percent of women in Africa and Asia work in the service sector, and less than 6 percent in industry (Ducommun 1980). Urban women work predominantly in the informal sector, not reported in labor statistics. Approximately half the female labor force in India is in the informal sector (Mazumdar 1976, reported in ICRW 1980), and for the same amount of work time as males in that sector they earn half as much income (Papdia 1980).

A major factor women report as influencing them to enter the labor market is economic need (Rivera 1979; Saffioti 1975). Whether a woman's entrance into the market labor force is through choice or necessity, there are future costs to the household in terms of the tradeoffs between economic and household welfare factors. The effect of market participation on income, and therefore expenditure on commodities such as food, is likely to be positive for the household diet. Popkin and Solon (1976) found Filipino women entering the work force increased weekly food expenditures by 1 to 5 percent. On the other hand, the time available for other aspects of food handling may be decreased in association with market labor, with negative effects on diet quality. There is some evidence of the negative effect of women's participation in market work in Asian countries on preschoolers' nutrient intake, breast-feeding, and child care (DaVanzo and Lee 1983; Popkin 1978). Evenson and King-Quizon (1978) found that only when Filipino women began to work in market production for more than six hours a day did household food production time decline. A study in Guatemala did not find a change in the time allocated to child care or breast-feeding when a woman left home to work (McGuire 1979). The

Guatemalan women did spend less time on food handling and household maintenance, but McGuire felt this was compensated for by greater efficiency in task performance.

The effects of woman's work in market activities on her nutritional status may be mediated by such factors as:

1. *The extent to which the woman's job supplements family income.* Women are typically restricted to lower-paying jobs, earn substantially less than males per unit of work time, and have little chance of promotion because of a system maintaining their low educational and skill levels (Singh 1977; World Bank 1979). Their earnings, therefore, may not always justify the time and welfare losses to household production. However, some studies have shown that under many circumstances, additional income from the woman's work outside the home is a benefit to the family that may well offset other welfare costs to the household (Evenson et al. 1979).

2. *The extent to which labor force participation takes time from household production activities.* When the labor market structure allows flexibility in working hours, as may be the case in the informal business sector or agriculture, labor force activities do not necessarily imply a decline in the woman's role at home (Evenson and King-Quizon 1978). DaVanzo and Lee (1983) show in Malaysia that employment in agriculture was not always compatible with home production, particularly with child care. Household diet would be expected to suffer where a woman's job involves long, inflexible hours.

3. *The extent to which other family members substitute time in home production activities.* Evidence indicates that older children, particularly girls, may substantially substitute in household work (Birdsall and McGreevey 1983; Jayme-Ho 1976; Pala 1979; Popkin and Solon 1976). While other household members may carry out a working mother's home production activities, the effect on household diet would depend on the quality of the substitution. Some evidence indicates that this substitution by children and others in the household does not appear to compensate for the woman's home production effort (Popkin and Solon 1976), particularly for food preparation (Ho 1979).

The effects of time allocation on maternal diet relative to the rest of the household may function directly through the dimension of time available for food activities already described. Also, female labor force participation is associated with changes in women's economic and social roles. The woman's increased economic contribution and changes in social status which may result would be expected to exert a positive effect on intrahousehold food allocation to her. In addition a woman's time and income allocation may affect her ability to use health and social services. Her use of prenatal care, family planning, nutrition services, and so on, are associated with health and nutritional benefits for herself and other household members. However, time constraints may be an important factor in underuse of these programs. Gopaldas et al. (1975) found this to be the factor contributing to poor participation by low-income women in a supplementary food distribution program. Similarly, the time and energy necessary for clinic attendance limited participation of African women in maternal-child health programs (Bornstein and Kreysler 1972).

Programs often demand time investments from women rather than helping them "make time" by teaching them to be more efficient and productive. An interesting exception has been the Women's Education Project in Upper Volta, which by introducing labor-saving technologies to create free time for education, inadvertently increased the time allocated to household tasks, such as meal preparation (McSweeney and Freedman 1980). Time allocation studies have consistently demonstrated the lack of free time common to low-income women, which must be taken into account in planning nutrition and health programs for women (Evenson and King-Quizon 1978; Farouk and Ali 1975; Popkin and Solon 1976).

HOUSEHOLD SIZE, PARITY, AND STRUCTURE

Household Size

Larger household size is frequently detrimental to the nutritional status of family members in low-income countries (Rao and Gopalan 1971; Wray and Aguirre 1969). For families with resource constraints, increased household size means fewer per capita resources, and the quantity and quality of the household's diet may suffer. A study in Colombia showed a significant drop in per capita food expenditure with increasing numbers of children in the family (Wray 1971). Possible countervailing forces are that economies of scale exist in large families, there is more labor for home production of foods, and older children may supplement household income. Some studies have shown that large household size may not necessarily have deleterious effects on income or food availability, since siblings may cause an increase in total family income that more than compensates for the additional cost, and they contribute to food gathering activities (Kelly et al. 1976; Russell 1976). In the situation of large family size and resource constraints, discrimination in intrahousehold food allocation may place females at greatest disadvantage (Florencio and Aligaen 1980).

Household size may affect maternal dietary needs in terms of the additional energy and time expenditure imposed on the mother to take care of more children and perhaps to assume roles outside the household (such as in the labor market). However, in large households, older (particularly female) children may also assume some of the household and child care activities.

Parity
Women of higher parity are more prone to anemia (Venkatachalam 1968) and lower weight-to-height ratios (Venkatachalam 1962). They are also at greater risk of pregnancy complications (toxemia, infection, hemorrhage, etc.), chronic ill health, and increased risk of such diseases as diabetes, cervical cancer, hypertension, and rheumatoid arthritis (Blair 1980), all of which may ultimately affect nutritional status. Women of larger low-income families are more likely to suffer illnesses through the facilitated exchange of disease agents through crowding (Cassel 1971). In addition they are less likely to have the income or time to seek medical assistance.

It is not only family size or parity which affects a woman's nutritional status but also the interval between pregnancies, which represents an important opportunity for the woman to replenish her nutrition stores. The repeated, closely spaced pregnancies associated with large family size have direct health and nutritional outcomes for the mother as well as her children (Wishik and Van der Vynkt 1975). Sequential cycles of pregnancy and lactation without a sufficient nonreproductive interval can lead to general maternal depletion, as shown by progressive weight loss and a prematurely aged appearance. Nutrient deficiencies leading to anemia, osteomalacia, edema, and enlarged goiter may also occur with repeated closely spaced pregnancies (Jelliffe and Maddocks 1964).

Family Structure
The structure of both nuclear and extended non-Western families has been characterized by exemplifying male supremacy, strong familialism, and inherent protective mechanisms for family members (Buvinić and Youssef 1978). Recent evidence has challenged these assumptions. An increasing number of households have female heads (Birdsall and McGreevey 1983; Buvinić and Youssef 1978); these may be widows, divorcees, women who are separated or abandoned, and single mothers. Women who are temporarily household heads through the job-related migration of husbands represent an important category, particularly in countries such as Yemen where a significant proportion of male household heads are employed in other Near East countries.

The rise in female family headship may be a corollary of economic development, which has fostered changes through urbanization, migration, and wage labor (Tinker 1976). The average percentage of potential household heads who are women is estimated to be 22 percent for sub-Saharan Africa, 20 percent for Central America and the Caribbean, 16 percent for North Africa and the Middle East, and 15 percent for South America (Buvinić and Youssef 1978). Exact national statistics are unavailable. The number of households at the poverty level headed by women is consistently higher than among other types of households (Elizaga 1970, reported in Buvinić and Youssef 1978; Merrick and Schmink 1983). Female household heads are likely to have to work out of need, and to suffer the same job and earning constraints faced by most other females. They are usually less educated and have fewer skills than male household heads. They also have fewer secondary workers to help bring in family income, less time for home production activities, and, in many cases, increased social disadvantages, according to the community's cultural norms (Merrick and Schmink 1983). The economic and social characteristics of female-headed households may therefore place serious constraints on the woman's ability to meet her own nutritional needs, as well as those of other household members.

However, not all types of households headed by women are similarly impoverished. It is important to differentiate such households according to why the male head is absent. Basson (1982) found Indonesian households headed by women because of husbands' employment-related migration had higher per capita incomes and higher levels of domestic productivity than did households with resident or weekend male heads. Members of such female-headed households are expected to enjoy a higher nutritional status.

New research also makes it increasingly apparent that the internal structure of the household may belie the ultimate focus of decision-making. More senior family members living in separate households often control decisions which affect the allocation of time, work activities, and resources within the household (Bauer 1981; Gulick and Gulick 1974). In addition obligations to family members outside the household may direct the allocation of scarce household resources to activities such as the production of a huge wedding feast, or to the support of relatives who have migrated to the city for work or education. Rural families regularly send supplies of rice, potatoes, onions, bread, cheese, and yogurt to relatives in the urban centers of Iran (Bauer 1981).

Studies on the power and authority of women are increasingly uncovering their important role in intradomestic (and perhaps inter-domestic) activities. While there are both presumptions and some research results which indicate that household structure is such that male members receive disproportionate amounts of household calories and nutrients, there is little empirical research on the advantages women enjoy in the actual preparing and distribution of food from the kitchen or their authority in allocation of resources within the household itself. At family gatherings in segregated societies, men may sit in privileged quarters enjoying high status foods like chicken, meat, and rice, but women can be observed in the kitchen consuming or saving choice portions for themselves, unnoticed by other family members (Beck 1978). At the same time cultural norms (discussed later) often dictate that men, not women, handle the purchasing of foods in markets and bazaars which are farther away from the household (Cain et al. 1979; Magnarella 1974).

Household composition also mediates a woman's position and authority within her own home. The division of labor and relative power of women vis à vis other family members is affected by the presence of in-laws or the spouses of husbands' older brothers in extended households. This is particularly noticeable in societies where early age at marriage places women in extended households at a young age. Young married women may carry increased burdens of labor for their mothers-in-law and other senior women, and may not attain the right to run their own households or control food resources and preparation until the departure of these older female kin (Friedl 1975; Hammond and Jablow 1976). In polygamous households, additional wives and children may constitute an economic drain on available capital or food resources. Conversely, they may contribute to household resources by participating in the labor market, increasing the home production of foods, or increasing time-use options by sharing child care and cooking responsibilities. In polygamous households in Zaire, wives may compete for the husband's attention by offering elaborate or expensive foods, to the detriment of their own and their children's diets (Tandberg 1980).

A woman's position in the household is also very much affected by life cycle and demographic changes. The young wife will eventually become a senior household member enjoying the rights of control over resources and labor allocations. One of the noticeable effects of urban industrial change has been an inversion of this life cycle effect (Bauer 1979; Makhlauf and Overmeyer 1978). Wives coming into marriges with increased knowledge and at older ages may have control over the organization of their own households and intrahousehold food distribution much sooner than in the past.

ENVIRONMENTAL CONDITIONS

Seasonal Variations

Rural populations in tropical environments of marked climatic seasonality have been estimated to number over one billion people, representing a high proportion of the very poor people in the world (Chambers 1979). Besides the more obvious impact of climatic seasonality on agricultural patterns, food supply, nutritional status, and disease prevalence, seasonal patterns have also been found in employment, income, migration, vital events, and government interventions (Chambers et al. 1979; Chen et al. 1979; Longhurst and Payne 1979; Schofield 1979). Seasonal factors negatively affecting nutritional status often occur at the same time. Studies of tropical farmers indicate the concurrence of seasonal food shortages, high demands for agricultural work, high morbidity and mortality, malnutrition, poor care for children, and financial indebtedness (Chambers et al. 1979). Because of their particular roles in such societies, these conditions may prove especially adverse for women.

The seasonal nature of family food availability in agrarian societies is predominantly caused by rainfall and cropping effects on food production. Food shortages occur more frequently in regions with a unimodal distribution of rainfall and a one-harvest system (Schofield 1979); erratic onset and distribution of rains throughout the growing season; and undiversified agricultural production (Annegers 1973). Annegers also finds seasonal infestations of locusts and birds and the lack of long-term food storage facilities to be major factors in regional differences in the severity of seasonal undernutrition. Inadequate household food stocks and high prices of staples coincide with the period of greatest food shortage in the agricultural cycle (Chen et al. 1979). The availability of irrigation, drought-resistant seed varieties, and food storage facilities can mitigate the effects of seasonal food availability. Adequate total availability of food to families requires either adequate employment opportunities to ensure a wage income sufficient for food purchases, or household control of food production resources (land, tools, labor). In Bangladesh landless mothers had lower average body weights and greater variance seasonally around the mean than did mothers in families with two acres of land or more (Chowdhury et al. 1978).

Seasonal changes in nutrient intake and nutritional status have been the subject of several reviews (Annegers 1973; Longhurst and Payne 1979). Nutrient availability has been shown to be seasonal in many regions, but the effect on adult females relative to other segments of the population is seldom reported. Reviewing a number of African studies, Schofield (1979) found a significant difference between the percentage fulfillment of caloric requirements in the wet (85 percent) and dry (92 percent) seasons. Seasonal fluctuation in nutrient intake in the Gambia ranged between 103 to 107 percent of requirements from November to January and 90 percent in June and July (R. H. Fox 1953). Other reviews have shown more severe deprivation in seasonal food intake (Annegers 1973).

Because of the seasonal nature of agriculture, work intensity is likely to fluctuate seasonally. Since women are often involved in agricultural production in tropical countries, the seasonal fluctuations in work loads may have an adverse impact on their other sphere of responsibility, home production, to the detriment of everyone's nutrition. Peak periods for women's work in the fields are normally at planting, harvesting, and postharvesting processing times, when the working day may average 15 hours (Palmer 1981); concurrently, food is commonly scarcest, more expensive, least varied, and least well prepared (Schofield 1979). During the peak agricultural season, Voltaic women spent 1.5 hours less each day on food preparation than during the dry season (Bleiberg et al. 1980). Since the increased food preparation during the dry season included preparation of food for sale, the direct impact on household and the women's nutrition is unclear.

Wage income opportunities are seasonal in certain areas and among certain socioeconomic groups. In much of Southeast and South Asia, for example, the seasonality of monsoon rice culture generates full employment only about two to three months of the year (Oshima 1971). In addition, agricultural wage rates drop during agricultural off-seasons

(Chen et al. 1979). Where family members engage in seasonal employment, the concomitant fluctuations in income and time allocation may affect total household diet. For the woman specifically, seasonal variation in her time and economic contribution to the household may be expected to influence the quantity and kinds of foods allocated to her relative to other household members through the income, time, and status variables already discussed.

Changes in energy expenditure and body weight have been linked to seasonal work patterns (Bleiberg et al. 1980; Brun et al. 1981). R. H. Fox (1953) measured levels of energy expenditure in the Gambia and showed that changes in body weight corresponded to patterns of farming activity and food availability. In this study the mean weights of adults showed very similar seasonal fluctuations. However, the weight differential between males and females in the dry and wet seasons (season of lowest body weight) was 12 and 20 pounds respectively, suggesting that the nutritional status of women was more susceptible than that of men to insult during deprivation periods. Similarly, a Ghanaian study reported average seasonal losses by adult men of 6.2 percent of body weight, compared to an average for females of 6.5 percent (Hunter 1967). Other studies have shown a seasonal effect on weight gain during pregnancy (Thomson et al. 1966). In Gambia, Whitehead and others (1978) found that during the wet season women in the last trimester of pregnancy lost an average of 1.4 kg. The average energy intakes of lactating women in the same population fell to less than 50 percent of recommended intake during the rains, reducing their capacity for lactation (Paul et al. 1979b).

A significant factor contributing to the seasonal stress of households is morbidity. It is well known that infections result in aberrations of nutrition balance, and conversely, that malnutrition increases susceptibility to infection and the severity of consequent disease (Scrimshaw 1975). The seasonal concurrence of food shortages and increased disease prevalence found in many parts of the world constitutes a high nutritional risk for the rural poor (Chambers 1979). Bradley (1981) delineates two major categories of seasonally variable diseases. In the majority, climatic events favor disease transmission at a certain season, and the progression from infection to manifest disease is short enough for clustering of cases. Less commonly, there are diseases where regulatory mechanisms defer the most disabling stages of illness to a particular season, such as with guinea worm. The main climatic factors determining disease cycles are rainfall and temperature (Chambers et al. 1979). Generally, the wet season is the time for a rise in the incidence of diarrheal disease, malaria, the guinea worm, and skin infections (Bray 1981; Chowdhury et al. 1978; Muller 1981; Porter 1981; Rowland et al. 1981). Chambers (1979) suggests that the stresses of seasonal disease are exacerbated by rural health services being at their least effective during the wet season, partly because of inadequate transportation and impassable roads.

Women are frequently at a disadvantage in the intrahousehold allocation of food, particularly when food supplies become inadequate during the hungry season. A further condition adverse for women and infants is the tendency documented in many countries for the birth rate to peak in the late rains and around harvest time (Becker and Sardar 1981; Dyson and Crook 1981; Mata 1978). The nutritional demands associated with concurrent pregnancy or lactation, heavy work loads, disease, and food shortages make women particularly vulnerable to these seasonal cycles.

The results of studies on seasonality and nutrition require cautious interpretation. Difficulty in interpreting the extent of nutritional imbalance in various seasons arises when dietary intakes are expressed as a percentage fulfillment of calculated requirements for a healthy reference population with a constant standard level of activity. However, since seasonally low dietary intake frequently coincides with increased disease incidence (Chambers et al. 1979) and energy expenditure (Chen et al. 1979; Thomson et al. 1966; Wilmsen 1978), nutritional needs will be markedly increased during this season. Reporting of dietary deficiency, particularly in the season of worst deprivation may therefore be underestimated.

Urban Residence

The location of household residence in specific rural or urban areas will affect the availability of food and health resources, labor opportunities, and vulnerability to disease and seasonal cycles. Broad-based changes in food availability, accessibility, storage, processing, preparation, and consumption are particularly associated with the processes of urbanization and modernization occurring with variable rapidity in low-income countries. From 1950 to 1975 the average proportion of the population in urban areas in Africa, Asia (except Japan), and Latin America grew from 16.7 percent to 28.0 percent, primarily from the natural increase of urban populations rather than through rural-urban migration (Preston 1979). Preston found urban growth has been fastest, other things being equal, where economic levels and economic growth rates are highest. Simultaneous changes in education and work opportunities, in access to health care, water supplies, family planning and other social services, and in social factors, such as the roles of women, are generally integral to economic growth and urbanization. The potential impact of these changes on food habits and nutritional status is considerable.

In urban areas, potential household income is greater than in rural areas, although the expenses of urban living are also higher (Reutlinger and Selowsky 1976). However, increased income is not necessarily positively associated with improved purchasing power or improved diet quality or quantity in urban areas. Evidence indicates, in fact, that a poor urban family may be nutritionally worse off than a poor rural family (Basta 1977). It is important to note that while urban health statistics generally look better than rural ones, the statistics for squatter and slum dwellers either are not included or the great discrepancies between low and middle/upper income groups counteract them. Basta (1977) reviews studies showing large differences in disease incidence and nutrient availability between low- and high-income urban groups and much smaller urban-rural differences.

A number of factors may contribute to the inadequate food availability and nutritional status of the low-income urban population. Food purchases depend on daily income, which necessitates the daily purchase of small quantities of food at higher unit prices. In addition, slum and shanty-town dwellers frequently lack access to central food markets and must depend on the limited range, quality, and higher prices of small shops and vendors (Hollinsteiner 1978). Time allocation to money-earning activities reduces the time available for food preparation and may encourage the use of ready-made or easy-to-prepare foods--usually more expensive and less nutritious than unprocessed alternatives. The high cost of fuel may also limit home preparation of food (Katona-Apte 1977b). The urban household does not usually have the advantage of home-produced foodstuffs. Not only is a continuous supply of cash a necessity for food purchases, but the reciprocal food arrangements between social or economic groups (e.g., landlords and tenants) often associated with harvest surpluses are lacking. Dietary choices of the urban household may be considerably influenced by such factors as media advertising or contact with modern health professionals. With initial adaptation to urban life styles (and increasingly, with the expansion of urban influences to the countryside) preferences for and access to status-producing foods also increase. The familiar jokes about American fast food and Coca Cola awaiting tourists in every country reflect the extent to which soft drinks, sweets, and other high prestige and low-nutrient density items are consumed by low-income and urban families--with potentially serious repercussions for nutrient intake and dental health.

However, in some countries, urban migrant food consumption may actually improve if assessed on year-round access to different food groups. For example, in urban Iran, low-income migrant households have access to wider varieties of fruits, vegetables, rice, and dairy products than do their rural counterparts. Many rural villages in Iran are cut off from other regions by heavy snows and poor transportation during those months in which their own crops and dairy products reach minimum levels (Bauer 1981). Some urban residents also have the advantages of refrigerated storage, greater access to health services--particularly quality services--and enjoy a more constant availability of water (Bauer 1981). Wolfe et al. (1980) found individuals with access to publicly or privately supplied internal water or wells have better health; city residence is more likely to be accompanied by such water supplies in low-income countries. Urban residence also means greater access to government agencies, programs providing information, and media sources of information (Akin et al. 1981; Basta 1977; Popkin and Solon 1976).

Urban women are generally undergoing great changes in their

economic and social options. Urban areas offer better employment opportunities for women and the potential income from market labor is usually greater. Changing concepts of family structure and factors such as migration in search of employment have given rise to female-headed households in both rural and urban areas. Selective male migration to urban areas, particularly in parts of Asia and Africa (Basta 1977; Preston 1979), may have a considerable impact on a number of factors affecting maternal diet and nutritional status. Not only are the women frequently left to assume work previously done by their husbands, but they are often called on to send food to them in urban areas.

The woman in a nuclear, extended, or single-parent household is usually the key person handling food purchase and preparation. How recently, and to what degree, a woman has adopted an urban life style will influence the expediency of her food-related decisions and her use of markets, transportation, credit systems, and health and social services. Food intake of the urban woman may be affected by the mechanisms already discussed in association with income, work, and household structure.

Related to urban residence and the expansion of urban influences and socioeconomic change in general is the extent to which development has radically changed traditional living environments. There is little research which assesses the effect of the destruction of forest areas or the sedentarization of hill tribes and pastoral nomads on the availability of traditional dietary items or adequate substitutes. As game and fish are destroyed, or households are encouraged to take up settled ways of life, attention is rarely given to retraining the population in agricultural methods or the use of foods more suitable to the new life style. Similarly, as rural households are faced with increasing forces of urbanization and development, we could expect to find large changes in diet and dietary needs. The ultimate effects of these changes on women's nutrition remains largely unknown.

EDUCATION AND INFORMATION

The terms *education* and *information* are used to include formal schooling, nonformal adult education, and knowledge informally acquired by the transmission processes and adaptive strategies which develop within different cultural contexts. Studies have focused predominantly on how formal education affects specific behavior patterns. Both general and specific nutrition education seems to improve household production of food, holding income constant (Chernichovsky 1978; Fiedler et al. 1978; Heller and Drake 1979).

Knowledge and information can affect household food intake in several ways. Education appears to increase the ability to absorb new ideas and use them for improved selection, allocation, and use of resources (Lockheed et al. 1980; T.W. Schultz 1975; Welch 1970, 1973). Education can affect the way households allocate their available income and time to food and other expenditures. It also influences the efficiency with which households store and prepare foods. Florencio and Smith (1969) found persons with more education are better able to produce a nutritious diet with less effort and fewer inputs, since they purchase, prepare, and distribute food more efficiently. Battad (1979) found women with higher levels of education bought more calories and protein per unit of food expenditure. Several researchers suggest that knowledge about proper food preparation and age- and sex-specific nutritional needs improves the final nutrient value and intrafamily allocation of foods (Berg 1973; Selowsky and Taylor 1973; Sharman 1970). However, little careful research has been conducted in this area.

In almost all developing countries there are sex-based disparities in access to education. A World Bank report (Haddad 1980) indicates that as an average for developing countries, 71.8 percent of 6- to 11-year-old males compared to 56.1 percent of females were enrolled in school in 1975 and 1977. In the 12-to-17 age group, 43.9 percent of males compared to 31.1 percent of females were enrolled. In regions such as Latin America and the Caribbean, sex-based disparities in school enrollment are minimal, whereas in many Asian, African, and Middle Eastern countries females are clearly at a disadvantage for receiving the benefits of formal education.

Educational opportunities for women are improving in some countries with processes of modernization and governmental commitments to altering the inequalities of schooling (McSweeney and Freedman 1980). Given the concomitant social changes in education, socioeconomic participation status, and income levels with development, the independent effects of these factors on women's nutrition are often difficult to separate. LeVine (1980) reviews evidence showing that women's schooling affects their fertility and infant and child mortality, independent of income, husband's education, and other factors attributable to the mother's external situation. One explanation LeVine offers for this phenomenon is that schooling promotes awareness of means-ends relationships in the environment and the capacity to use this awareness in new contexts. A woman with more education is therefore more likely to see the relationship between diet and health. Whether this knowledge has the potential to alter dietary choices depends on economic and cultural constraints. In some instances benefits may have to be perceived by household members other than just the woman in order for changes in food production, buying, storage, preparation, allocation, or consumption to occur.

A woman's nutritional status is influenced by disease incidence which is in turn associated with knowledge of disease processes. Knowledge may affect whether a woman boils the drinking water, adequately cleans cooking utensils, or effectively disposes of human waste (Okediji 1975). Knowledge also affects use of health services (Akin et al. 1981), which can have an important effect on nutritional and health status during pregnancy, pregnancy outcome, family planning, and other health-related practices. Education and information affects women's work potential, income-generating capacity, social status, and use of health and social service programs. The impacts of these factors on women's nutrition are discussed in other sections.

Informal sources of information, such as government programs, media campaigns, and community leaders, have important effects on women's nutritional practices (Mernissi 1978). In some households, illiterate mothers receive health-related information via their school-age children who either read about health and nutrition in their school books or, in some cases, are directed by their teachers to relay certain kinds of information to their parents (Bauer 1981). Rogers and Kincaid (1981) have extensively analyzed the role of key women in Korean village mothers clubs who serve as role models and sources of information on family planning for other, less informed women in the village. These sources of information, however, are much harder to record and analyze than formal education. A number of studies have correlated media exposure to women's knowledge and attitudes about various topics (R.H. Fox 1953). Rural Iranian women with no access to television programming, nevertheless, displayed a surprising degree of knowledge on health issues and women's rights which had been broadcast on radio programs during the late 1970s (Bauer 1981).

CULTURAL DETERMINANTS

Cultural factors are important in conditioning the persistence of food habits and preferences, as are related factors such as women's work, household division of labor, age at marriage, and the tendency to bear large numbers of children. The direct and indirect effects of cultural mechanisms operating on nutrition behavior are too often overlooked.

Cultural systems impose restrictions on the consumption of certain foods, and these food taboos and beliefs very frequently affect women or young children (Jelliffe and Jelliffe 1967). For example, O'Laughlin (1974) has analyzed the conditions dictating the restriction of chicken consumption to male members of Mbum society. Documented food taboos characteristically involve the prohibition of protein foods for pregnant and lactating women (Ayres 1967; Bolton 1972; Katona-Apte 1977a, b; Richards 1939; Valdecañas 1971; Wilson 1978). Kusin et al. (1979) report that 10 to 15 percent of mothers interviewed in East Java observe food restrictions during pregnancy and lactation. However, in food taboo research, there is little discussion of the imposition or observation of these cyclical food restrictions during less critical stages of a woman's life cycle or of their nutritional impact--little research has shown that these taboos do affect diet during other phases of the life cycle. Many customs involving the consumption of special foods for women, for example, occur during very limited periods of time--such as during or after childbirth and at the consummation of the first marriage (Kendall 1968). In addition, in many traditional societies the intake of animal foods such as chicken, goats, and pigs is always limited to ritual or festive occasions.

Disproportionate distribution of food and nutrients within the household in favor of males may be an important factor contributing to the sex bias in nutritional status found in many societies. As discussed in the section on economics, there is some evidence that food distribution within the family may relate to the economic contribution of household members, with women generally contributing less income and therefore receiving less food than men. Discrimination against females in infrahousehold food allocation in many societies is related to their inferior status role and work opportunities. This is one explanation Chen et al. (1981) offer for rural Bangladesh where males' calorie consumption exceeds females' by 29 percent in the childbearing age group. Male daily protein intake in the same age group was 73.6 gm compared to 58.8 for females. The caloric differential remains substantial when adjusted for body weight and the calorie demands of pregnancy and lactation. In a study of Filipino households, Valenzuela et al. (1979) showed that the mean nutrient adequacy ratio and diet rating of fathers were generally higher than those of mothers, and were significant for protein and vitamin C.

Not only do cultures have preferred uses for foods and status foods, but they also have images of body types that denote health and well-being. In some societies rice has prestige over other carbohydrate foods like wheat or yams; and in these societies the more highly refined and polished (and the less nutritious) the rice is, the more highly valued it is. "Hot" and "cold" designations for foods often direct the preparation and consumption of foods during the different stages of women's childbearing years and during periods of illnesses. Researchers have generally found little consistency in the use of these categories even within the same culture.

In many parts of Asia, Africa, and the Middle East, rotundness has traditionally indicated health and even beauty (Richards 1939). In Iran, women in low-income urban areas attempt to gain weight soon after marriage to comply with this male preference. The health dangers involved in obesity and large weight gains are well documented. Similarly, cultural preferences regulate other practices related to health and nutrition--such as early age at marriage and social expectations for large family size. In cultures where women marry young and are encouraged to produce children while still in their early teens, a young woman's growth and long-term health prospects are strained by pregnancy during the period of her own rapid growth. In addition, most societies restrict the information which young, pubescent females have about their own bodily functions and needs (Paul 1974).

Occasionally, food preferences and health practices are rationalized in religious terms. Sanctions against particular foods (pork in the case of Islam) can be especially strong. Concepts of ritual cleanliness may also have nutritional and health repercussions. In societies where notions of periodic female uncleanliness prevail, the work roles of women are interrupted each month. These concepts of cleanliness associated with religious beliefs may bear little relation to biological conceptions of the causes of uncleanliness or disease.

The ethnographic, anthropological observation and reporting of interesting peculiarities in the use of food and in health practices is becoming less frequent as food preferences among remote groups change toward the urban, industrial norms of their respective nations and as formal education expands. Urban influences bring new food choices and the resources with which to acquire them, both of which tend to standardize preferences for various foods. In many instances, increasing change in and destruction of native habitats have meant subsequent reductions in availability of traditional foodstuffs and forced dietary change.

Cultural norms or preferences are the products of social and ecological factors interacting over time. In effect the concept of cultural preferences summarizes the effect of social interaction and social networks within select environments on the preferences of individuals and households. Research on women's status and roles in developing countries has documented how women's failure to seek extradomestic employment and their restriction to household domains is partly because these are considered female status behaviors within that group or culture (el-Messiri 1978; Jacobson 1978; Papanek 1973; Remy 1975; Youssef 1974). Women have been constrained to bear large families because of pressure from their neighbors and in-laws to produce many children, especially sons. Such behaviors indicate that those things which symbolized cultural status in the past often change very slowly.

The household's relationship to neighborhood and community is reflected in the degree to which it is willing to deviate from older cultural expectations in the use of food, or in other behaviors. Rogers and Kincaid (1980), for example, have explained women's changing rates of adopting contraception in Korea by analyzing the composition of their social networks. After a certain number of women in a network have been using a particular method of contraception, other women in that group are more likely to adopt the same method of family planning. In any program of nutrition intervention, it will be important to assess the preferences shared by other households with whom women and their families maintain close contact and who provide the potential environment for supporting change in cultural expectations.

Chapter 5
Summary: Significance, Patterns, and Determinants

Research and programming in women's nutrition has generally examined women within the context of their childbearing role. The areas of focus have been the consequences of women's nutritional status and diet during pregnancy and lactation for the infant's viability and health. While this concern for the health of forthcoming generations is very important, it is equally critical to establish a broader perspective for examining women as a nutritionally vulnerable group in their own right. Women fulfill unique social, economic, and cultural roles which affect their nutritional vulnerability in addition to their biological roles; the nutritional implications of these roles affect not only women's sense of health and well-being, but also the movement of communities towards national development goals.

In examining the important consequences of women's nutritional status and diet during the reproductive years, research has tended to concentrate on the functional outcome of moderate and severe malnutrition, while little is still known about the effects of marginal malnutrition. In a number of studies, supplemental calorie and/or protein intake during pregnancy by women at risk of producing low birth weight babies has been associated with increased infant birth weight. The degree to which prenatal supplementation affects birth weight varies considerably between studies, and the specifics of optimal supplementation remain to be identified. The mechanisms by which nutrition during pregnancy affects human fetal growth must be clarified. However, evidence is such that underweight women should be encouraged to increase their dietary intake during pregnancy as a means toward improving pregnancy outcome. Evidence also suggests that women's preconception nutritional status affects birth weight and efforts to improve it should begin in childhood.

Evidence of a link between women's nutritional status and their fertility remains controversial. At this stage, several of the biological components determining fertility such as age at menopause, regularity of ovulation, and the probability of intrauterine mortality appear to be little influenced by nutritional status. There is more evidence to suggest a small, although possibly insignificant fertility effect of improved nutritional status on lowering the age at menarche and shortening the period of lactational amenorrhea. This, however, should not be construed by population planners as a reason for not improving women's nutritional status for fear of increasing their fertility. The possibly differential effects of acute versus chronic malnutrition on fertility remain to be clarified.

Women's nutritional status has been examined in relation to lactation performance. Calorie intake may have an important influence on breast milk quantity with reduced intakes rapidly affecting milk output and dietary supplementation increasing yields. In addition a woman's nutritional status prior to and during pregnancy may influence her milk yield. Some evidence indicates that dietary intake affects the quality of breast milk, particularly the amino acid pattern, the fatty acids, and water-soluble vitamin content. It is unclear, however, whether increasing certain nutrients in breast milk by supplementation improves the infants' nutritional status. There is insufficient evidence to date to draw any conclusions about the effects of a woman's nutritional status on the length of time she is able to lactate.

Among women in low-income countries, one of the important functional consequences of nutritional status is morbidity. Reliable information on patterns of disease is unattainable on a country-wide basis for most nations, and the health data that exist are frequently not sex-disaggregated. It is generally not possible to distinguish the diseases that may specifically affect women. Poor nutritional status increases the susceptibility to and the severity of infections, as well as the functional effects of infectious diseases, which are the major causes of morbidity in low-income countries. The nature and prevalence of chronic diseases thought to have a nutritional component in their etiology has been studied extensively in industrialized nations, but little in low-income countries. Evidence indicates women are at higher risk than men for developing hypertension, diabetes mellitus, and obesity. Of the nutritional diseases, anemia is the most important to affect women, leading to diverse physiological and psychological sequelae. About half the nonpregnant women, and nearly two-thirds of the pregnant women in low-income countries have hemoglobin concentrations indicating anemia.

Studies of the effects of nutrition on labor productivity have been conducted primarily on men, and it is unclear whether the results can be generalized to women who generally work under very different conditions. Poor nutritional status appears to decrease the total time a person can work, the intensity of that work, and the kind of work selected. Variations in iron status and intake may be a more significant nutritional determinant of labor productivity than variations in energy intake. The productivity implications of nutrition are particularly important to women who have higher incidences of iron deficiency anemia than males. Studies also indicate that women's work time and productivity do not significantly alter during pregnancy and lactation when their nutritional needs are highest.

Comprehensive data on women's nutritional status in developing countries are severely lacking. What information exists is based primarily on very small samples and is generally limited to data on pregnant and lactating women. While it is impossible to make broad generalizations, women (and men) in many of the populations studied have deficient diets, while in some of the newly Westernized societies, people suffer problems of dietary excesses. Deficient caloric intake is common among nonpregnant and lactating women. Studies indicate that in many societies women consume a smaller percentage of their recommended daily intake than men. Protein intakes appear to be more adequate than caloric intakes, but women often consume lower quality protein than men. Calcium and iron are women's most serious common micronutrient deficiencies. Inadequate dietary intakes are reflected in anthropometric and biochemical measures of nutritional status, frequently below reference standards, though not as low as the magnitude of dietary deficiencies would suggest.

In addition to the biological indications of women's nutritional status, socioeconomic and cultural factors also provide important, although less direct information about women's nutritional risk in developing countries. Studies have focused primarily on the effects of these factors on the household diet generally, and the specific effects on women's nutrition require clarification. Households facing income and time constraints, with large numbers of children, low education levels, and poor access to information, or subject to a poor urban environment or seasonal variations in food supply, work, and disease will be at greater nutritional risk. We argue that these conditions frequently place the woman of the household at higher nutritional risk, either directly or indirectly, than her male counterpart.

Income-generating activities are often not as readily available or socially acceptable for women, and are less remunerative than for men. Economic contribution to the household has important links to relative equality, decision making, and the control and distribution of resources such as food. Women in developing countries commonly work longer hours per day than men and engage in energy-intensive, low-technology work, such that the nutritional demands of their work and time may be significant. The time constraints of women have been shown to be an important factor in their underuse of health service and nutrition programs. The large household size common to families in many developing countries places a woman at nutritional risk from the biological demands of pregnancy and lactation. Household size also affects dietary needs on account of the additional time and energy expenditure imposed on the mother to take care of the children, and perhaps to assume economic roles outside the household. There are an increasing number of female-headed households in developing countries whose economic and social characteristics place serious constraints on the woman's ability to meet her own nutritional needs, as well as those of other members of the household.

The effect of seasonality on diet and nutritional status is intimately bound up with such factors as seasonal patterns in agriculture, work, energy expenditure, and disease. During periods of deprivation, women's body weights have been shown to be more adversely affected than males, with adverse effects on weight gain during pregnancy and lactation ability. Women are at particular disadvantage in the intrahousehold allocation of food during the hungry season. For the increasing number of newly urbanized women, their diets and nutritional status will be linked to the adaptation to changes in social and economic options, and the use of markets, services, and new food and resource choices. Both general education and specific nutrition education seem to improve household food production, and thus nutritional status. In many developing countries women are at a distinct disadvantage for receiving the benefits of formal education. In some societies, a number of cultural determinants adversely affect women's nutritional status, such as imposing restrictions on the consumption of certain foods, particularly during pregnancy and lactation; the disproportionate distribution of food in favor of male household members; and women eating last and least at a meal. Finally, on a physiological level, studies indicate that in many societies women appear to be more overworked than males. Women may also be at greater risk of infectious disease since as mothers they are in contact with ill family members. Women deserve special attention in this regard since the nutritional demands of others may exacerbate the already marginal nutritional status, or be compounded by the simultaneously high nutritional demands of pregnancy or lactation. Women of childbearing age in developing countries spend the majority of their time either pregnant or lactating, and dietary studies show they rarely meet their additional nutritional needs during these times.

A broad range of factors encompasses many aspects of a woman's existence that can affect her nutritional status. In view of the tremendous economic, time, and socio-cultural constraints women face, in addition to the biological demands of childbearing, it is clear that women require higher priority consideration by nutrition and development planners than they have hitherto received.

Chapter 6
Programs

In Chapter 5 we discussed a broad range of factors which collectively determine the nutritional status of women in developing countries. These determinants encompass many aspects of a woman's existence. Any changes in any of these factors will have some effect on a woman's health and nutrition. In the following section, we discuss the impacts on nutritional status of planned changes in some of the determining factors. We begin by reviewing nutrition intervention programs--how they can theoretically affect women's nutritional status, what evaluations have shown about their actual impacts, and how such programs can be more carefully designed to take into consideration the special situations of women in developing countries. In a similar manner, we then review the impact of primary health care programs, and, finally, the impacts on maternal nutritional status, theoretical and actual, of general development programs.

NUTRITION INTERVENTION PROGRAMS

A wide variety of programs to improve nutritional status in developing countries has been initiated. Most nutritionists and program planners view children as the group most vulnerable to malnutrition and the vast majority of nutrition intervention programs have focused on improving the nutritional status of infants and children. Women's nutritional status has been of concern primarily as it relates to their ability to produce healthy offspring. Nutrition intervention programs for women have focused almost exclusively on pregnant and lactating women, or on mothers of small children. Intervention programs generally do not address the long-term needs of women throughout their life cycle nor nutritional needs related to nonchild rearing functions.

Of the sample of 180 primary health service projects in developing countries surveyed by the American Public Health Association (1977), 90 percent offered some form of nutrition service with 74 percent working actively toward definite nutrition objectives. In only 15 percent, however, were mothers (not women in general) specifically identified as a target population. Similarly, in the preschool nutrition intervention programs reviewed by the Harvard Institute for International Development (Austin et al. 1978b), only one-third of those programs providing food supplementation specifically included pregnant and lactating women. Other programs provide services to the family or community as a whole, but there is little information available on the extent to which women receive these services, or to what extent they benefit from them.

Food Supplementation Programs

Food supplementation programs are a common nutrition intervention strategy in developing countries. The vast majority have been directed at improving the nutritional status of children and have included pregnant and lactating women as participants only to the extent that improving maternal nutritional status will improve children's health and nutrition (Beaton and Ghassemi 1983). Programs which have provided supplements to the entire family (such as food-for-work programs) have either not been evaluated in terms of nutritional impact, or have not specifically investigated the impact on women. There have been few evaluations of programs which supplement the diets of pregnant and lactating women. The evaluations highlight the emphasis on women as childbearers by evaluating maternal supplementation programs only in terms of their impact on pregnancy outcome and lactation behavior, and not in terms of their impact on women's long-term nutritional status throughout the life cycle. Indicators of program success have included improvements in birth weight and decline in infant mortality rates. Very little information is available on the portion of the supplement actually consumed by the woman, whether it is an addition to the normal diet or whether it acts as a substitute, and whether programs are successful in reaching the most undernourished women. No information could be found on the postpregnancy impact of supplementation on indicators of maternal nutritional status such as postpregnancy weight and iron status.

One of the better known field studies which reports the impact of maternal supplementation on mother's nutritional status took place in Guatemala under the auspices of the Institute of Nutrition of Central America and Panama (INCAP) (see Delgado et al. 1977, 1979; Habicht et al. 1973; Lechtig et al. 1975b). Although the objective of the study was to determine the impact of maternal supplementation on pregnancy outcome, some information on maternal nutritional status is also reported. The unsupplemented daily intake of pregnant women in the four rural villages averaged 1,500 calories and 40 grams of protein. Supplements were of two forms: a calorie and protein rich gruel (atole) and a beverage (frescoe) which contained one-third as many calories as the atole and no protein; both included vitamin and mineral supplements. The supplements, available twice a day, were to be consumed at the distribution center. Acceptance of the supplement was voluntary and the amount consumed was unrestricted but recorded daily. Dietary recalls were conducted prior to initiation of the program and at three times during the pregnancy. There appeared to be a negative but insignificant correlation between the amount of supplement and the home dietary intake, indicating that the supplement did not substitute, to any great extent, for other foods normally in the diet. For the purpose of analysis, participants were grouped according to the level of supplemental calories consumed during their pregnancy. Of those women consuming more than 20,000 calories of the supplement during their pregnancies, the mean caloric intake increased by 235 calories per day, or approximately 9 percent of their daily requirement. There were no differences between the groups in maternal height, age, parity, and weight at the end of the first trimester. However, members of the high supplement group were of a lower socioeconomic status and reported more days of illness during pregnancy than did members of the low supplement group. Since it was not the intent of the study to determine the optimal method of providing supplements to women, other factors which may have influenced the level of participation (such as distance to the distribution center and work load) were not investigated. Also, no follow-up information was presented which could be used to determine whether the supplement had any long-term effects on maternal health and nutritional status.

The impact on pregnancy outcome and child growth of two different types of supplementation programs was investigated in Mexico (Chávez and Martínez 1975; Chávez et al., 1980). One of the programs was a food-for-work program which provided monthly supplemental foods (maize, beans, meat, fish) for the entire family (equivalent to 6,000 calories a day per family) and an additional ration of powdered milk only to pregnant women. The second program distributed a supplement of milk powder only to pregnant women and children. No information is available on whether this supplement was taken home or consumed at the distribution site. The food-for-work program did not produce any long-term change in family caloric intake since it appears that the supplemental foods were substituted for foods normally in the home diet. Even though an additional supplement was provided for women, there was no change in the intrafamilial distribution of calories, indicating that the woman's supplement was shared among all family members. The second supplemental feeding program did show a significant increase in the mean caloric intake of the supplemented women versus comparable controls (from 1,960 calories per day to 2,410 calories per day) with a corresponding increase in weight gain during pregnancy and an increase in birth weight. Curiously, the supposed increase in caloric intake of the experimental group over the controls (450 cal per day) was larger than the supplement itself (250 cal per day). The authors attribute this to increased appetite among the supplemented women because of their improved feelings of well-being, and greater activity. Differences in initial intakes between the two groups and errors in dietary recall methodology are also likely explanations, but are not explored in the report.

An extensively documented large-scale maternal and child nutritional program was carried out in India as part of Project Poshak (Gopaldas et al. 1975). Pregnant and lactating women were given a weekly take-home supplement of instant corn soy milk equivalent to 754 calories and 38 grams of protein daily. The dietary impact on the women participants was minimal. Pregnant women consumed only one-tenth of their ration, increasing their caloric consumption by less than 100 calories per day. Lactating women consumed one-fourth of their ration and increased their caloric intake by 200 calories per day. Further information on the program's impact on nutritional status is not available. Collecting birth weight data appeared to be impossible because of the high incidence of home births, and clinical signs and morbidity data were difficult to collect because of the reluctance of women to be examined by male doctors. The authors conclude that the supplement probably had only a marginal effect on the women's nutritional status, primarily because their intake of calories and protein was already high. Even after supplementation, however, the diets were still deficient in vitamins A and C and calcium, suggesting that a simple vitamin and mineral supplement would have been more appropriate and less costly.

One of the few relatively long-term supplementation programs took place in Taiwan (McDonald et al. c.1980). Low-income rural women who were considered marginally malnourished (with an average daily intake of 1,400 calories and 40 grams of protein) were supplemented continuously from the birth of one child through their next pregnancy and period of lactation. The supplement was distributed twice daily at a feeding station and efforts were made to deliver it to working women unable to come to the distribution point. The daily supplement provided 800 calories and 40 grams of protein and its impact on the participating mothers was compared with a group of controls who received an 80-calorie a day supplement. Although the methods used to measure the amount of the supplement the women actually consumed and their total dietary intake were not highly accurate, the authors conclude that, following supplementation, the total daily calorie and protein intake of the experimental group was higher than that of the control group. However, there were no significant differences between the two groups in mean birth weights of the second infants or in the percentage of low birth weight infants. Curiously, maternal caloric intake was significantly correlated with birth weight only for the control group. The authors suggest that these results may relate to a threshold effect.

A supplementation program to improve the lactational

performance of Gambian mothers contained some information on the supplement's intermediate effects on the mother's nutritional status (Prentice et al. 1980). Baseline data collected over the year preceding the start of the program revealed that the mean caloric intake of lactating women ranged from 40 to 60 percent of the recommended level, depending on the season. A supplement, consisting of locally prepared biscuits and supplying between 950 and 1,100 calories per day was distributed six times a week. Measurements of total intake before and after the program revealed an increase in the mean caloric intake from 1,568 to 2,291 calories and a reduction in the seasonal intake variation. Home food intake decreased by only 107 calories a day, indicating a rather low rate of substitution of the supplement for foods already in the home diet. The supplemented women were one to two kg heavier throughout the period of lactation, although they still lost weight during the preharvest hungry season.

Supplemental feeding programs which rely on the supplement's being consumed in the home must consider that, although the supplement may be designated for one or more specific family members, it usually will be shared by the entire household. A maternal supplementation program in Colombia attempted to address this problem by providing a supplement for the entire family (Mora et al. 1979). Beginning with the third trimester of pregnancy, a weekly supplement was distributed to participating families which provided 856 calories and 38 grams of protein daily per family member. Dietary recalls of the intake of the pregnant women revealed that their mean daily intake was increased by only 155 calories and 20 grams of protein. It appears that either a considerable amount of substitution occurred, some family members consumed more than their calculated ration, or it was sold.

Another family supplementation program carried out in Peru (Baertl et al. 1970) provided two forms of white wheat noodles over a five-year period to families with young children or pregnant and lactating women. The amount of supplement was determined on the basis of family size and provided a theoretical addition of 250 calories and either 7.5 or 12.5 grams of protein per family member. It is not clear from the report how actual consumption of the supplement was measured. The authors suggest that the supplement was substituted to a great extent for the cassava and sweet potatoes already in the diet, especially among adults. Determination of the supplement's impact on the nutritional status of adult women was confounded by the fact that anthropometric measurements of women in the control and experimental villages were not initially identical. The heights and weights of adult women in all groups increased, suggesting that the supplement had a limited, if any, effect. The authors suggest that the result relates to a high degree of substitution of the supplement for other foods.

A few studies have investigated the factors affecting the success (or lack of it) of supplementation programs in improving the nutritional status of the target women. Participation rates were studied most extensively in Project Poshak in India (Gopaldas et al. 1975). In the project's initial exploratory phase, participation was very low among pregnant women. The authors attribute this to a tradition of not announcing one's pregnancy and to the belief that a large fetus made for a more difficult delivery. Lactating women were much more likely to participate, especially tribal women, women whose husbands were illiterate, and those who were exposed to a greater number of nutrition education sessions. The sample of pregnant participants was too small to draw any conclusions about factors influencing participation. A more thorough investigation of families with either eligible children or mothers found participation lower among families living more than 3 km from the distribution point, the landless, and large landowners. Families in small villages had higher participation rates. Participation also increased with family size, decreasing income, and eligibility of both mother and child. In a later phase of the project, when it was expanded and conducted as an adjunct to a health care program, participation rates were higher among population served by a satellite health clinic staffed only by an auxiliary nurse midwife (ANM) than among populations served by a comprehensive primary health clinic staffed by a number of professional and paraprofessional health workers. The authors conclude that the single ANM had more time to devote to the program.

Rao and Vijayaraghavan (1976) also found that distance affects participation in a food supplementation program. In their study, being more than five kilometers from the distribution center was negatively associated with participation. This study also estimated the extent of sharing the supplement with noneligible family members. An average of 72 percent of participating households admitted to some sharing; the figure was 63 percent when the eligible family member was a child and 82 percent when the mother was the one eligible for the supplement. The supplement was most commonly shared with children two to six years old and never with adult men. However, the amount of the supplement shared with other family members was not determined.

In the study by Chávez et al. (1980) in Mexico discussed earlier, two supplemental feeding programs were compared on the basis of their impact on nutritional status. Although the programs were not designed for comparison and therefore the populations were not necessarily comparable, the authors conclude that the greater success of the second program (supplementing the diet of pregnant women with powdered milk) came from better targeting and because the powdered milk could not easily be substituted for food normally consumed.

Table 13 is a summary of some of the more important characteristics of the programs reviewed above, listed in order of decreasing success in terms of impact on women's dietary intake. Before any general conclusions can be drawn from these studies, several warnings are in order. First of all, the success of any intervention program is highly dependent on local conditions. It cannot be assumed that what works in one country or even in one region within a country can be applied successfully elsewhere. Similarly, a program unsuccessful in one area may be successful somewhere else. Thus, making sweeping generalizations about factors affecting the success of nutrition programs is risky and such generalizations should always be considered in light of current local conditions. Second, all the programs reviewed above involved supplementaton of pregnant or lactating women. Probably such women are more highly motivated to improve their nutritional status than nonpregnant, nonlactating women. Factors linked with success in improving the nutritional status of the former group may not have the same degree of impact on the nutritional status of the latter group.

On-site programs seem generally more effective in improving maternal dietary intake than take-home programs. Substitution for foods normally in the home diet seems minimal and sharing the supplement with other family members is negligible in on-site supplementation. However, on-site programs are generally more expensive to operate than are equivalent take-home programs. It may also be difficult for the neediest of women, many of whom work outside the home in addition to performing all household chores, to find the time to make a daily (or twice daily) trip to the distribution center. As the Taiwan study indicates, a take-home program can be successful if a strong outreach component can deliver the supplement to women unable to pick up their ration themselves. Take-home programs appear more effective when the form of the supplement is somewhat different from foods normally consumed by the family. This may reduce the magnitude of sharing with noneligible family members. Another apparent characteristic of successful take-home programs is the frequency of distribution; more frequent distribution is associated with more effective programs.

Maternal supplementation programs which provide a ration for each family member appear to have only limited success. These programs generally provide food acceptable to the entire family and it may be that, because women are generally the last to eat at any meal, they actually consume much less than their alloted ration. Also, it is more likely that extensive substitution takes place when the supplement consists of common local foods. The only family supplementation program which seemed somewhat successful was the program in Bogotá in which only families with malnourished children were eligible. Other programs distributed the supplement to all families in the community regardless of nutritional need.

Targeting is an important issue to be considered in program development. With the exception of the Bogotá program, no other program targeted the supplement to women according to their current nutritional status. (The Taiwan study did not indicate whether all women in the study villages were marginally malnourished or whether only those who met certain criteria were eligible for the supplement.) Such targeting should reduce the costs of a supplemental feeding program and, by distributing food only to those who need it most, should improve the success rate. However, targeting requires additional administrative effort, the cost of which may (depending on the complexity of criteria) outweigh the savings. The value of targeting will depend on the prevalence of nutritional problems in an area. If 90 percent of women are nutritionally deficient, then targeting will not generate significant savings.

The lack of success in improving nutritional status in Project Poshak highlights the need to consider the quantity and quality of foods currently consumed by women when planning a supplementation program. If, as in the case of Project Poshak, the study population's diets are nearly adequate in calories and protein but deficient in vitamins and minerals, then supplementation with vitamin and mineral rich foods or vitamin supplements would be more appropriate and cheaper than caloric supplementation.

Nutrition Education Programs

Nutrition education programs are a well-known form of nutrition intervention: 88 percent of health care projects surveyed by the American Public Health Association contained a nutrition education component (APHA 1977) and 91 percent of the preschool nutrition intervention programs surveyed by the Harvard Institute for International Development (Austin et al. 1978b) provided nutrition education. The overall objective of these programs is to improve the maldistribution of food based on inadequate knowledge, presuming overall adequate food resources. Zeitlin and Formacion (1981) report on a study in India which demonstrated that even among families whose total food resources met or exceeded total needs, mean caloric intakes of family members of certain ages (notably children less than two and teenagers) fell below recommended levels.

While a majority of nutrition education programs have been designed to improve the nutritional status of children specifically, a good number have dealt with improving overall household diet. Since women are generally responsible for food preparation (as well as food production in many agricultural societies), nutrition education programs have generally been directed at them. The impact of such programs on women's nutritional status could be substantial. Nutrition education programs attempt to change knowledge and attitudes about certain of the immediate determinants of nutritional status. Programs to increase knowledge about home production, food purchasing, storage, and preparation can increase the quantity and quality of food available to the household. Other programs which strive to change inappropriate food beliefs and taboos or increase knowledge of the differing nutritional needs of different family members may improve intrahousehold food distribution.

Evaluations of the effectiveness of nutrition education programs in accomplishing these changes in knowledge and behaviors and thus improving women's status have been limited (Leslie 1977; USAID 1976;

Whitehead 1970; Zeitlin and Formacion 1981). Nutrition education programs are often only one component of a comprehensive health care program and it becomes extremely difficult to measure changes in behavior; most evaluations have concentrated on measuring only changes in knowledge and attitudes. In addition, behavior changes have rarely been related to long-term changes in nutritional status. Finally, since the emphasis of many nutrition education programs has been on improving child nutritional status, evaluations which consider the impact on women's nutritional status are rare.

Leslie (1977) reviewed evaluations of several mass media nutrition education programs, two of which had a potential impact on women's nutritional status. A radio and poster program in Ecuador addressed, among other subjects, protein calorie malnutrition, iodine deficiency, and breast-feeding. Surveys taken before and after completion of the program revealed an increased knowledge of protein sources among those who were aware of the campaign compared to those unaware of the campaign. However, even the latter group showed an increase in knowledge over their baseline levels, which Leslie attributed to a "multiplier effect" of the passing on of information. A similar improvement occurred in the percentage of respondents thinking breast milk was the best food for infants. A positive impact on behavior was demonstrated by an increased consumption of iodized salt, measured both by the survey and by monitoring sales. However, program impact appeared to wear off after broadcasting became less frequent.

An evaluation of a radio and print program in Korea (Leslie 1977) demonstrated wide outreach (92 percent of urban and 87 percent of rural subjects interviewed had been exposed to the radio broadcast) and a possible impact on knowledge. Fifty-three percent of those interviewed remembered advice to eat a balanced diet and 20 percent were able to name specific nutrients contained in items of different food groups. However, since the evaluation used no controls and collected no baseline data, it is impossible to measure changes in knowledge or to attribute the knowledge of the respondents to the nutrition education program.

A small but innovative nutrition education program on a plantation in Guatemala (Colle and Fernández de Colle 1978) used a series of dramatic nutrition education segments recorded on audio cassettes and played daily for three weeks at the outdoor public laundry, visited almost daily by women of the plantation. A survey of 40 plantation women and 10 control women from a neighboring plantation who did not receive the education program revealed that those who listened daily to the tapes had a higher level of knowledge than did occasional listeners, who also scored higher than the controls. Effects on behavior were demonstrated by the fact that 70 percent of the sample had memorized a special Incaparina recipe given on one of the tapes and 58 percent had tried the recipe.

After realizing that few nutrition education programs are adequately evaluated (Whitehead 1970), USAID (1976) developed a field guide for evaluating nutrition education projects and field tested the method on a number of projects, two of which were directed at improving women's general nutrition awareness. One was a series of formal nutrition classes offered to urban homemakers in Bogotá, Colombia. Dietary recalls were conducted at the beginning and end of the series and six months following completion; recalls were compared with a similar group of controls. At the end of the series of classes, participants had a significant improvement in their consumption of milk and vegetables. However, the improvement was not sustained; six months after completion of the classes, there was no significant difference in consumption by participants and controls. The evaluation method being tested included an evaluation of costs. The project was estimated to cost $4.25 per student and $19.25 per student who improved her intake on completion of the class. There was no accounting, however, for possible improvements in the diets of other household members (Shaw 1979, as quoted in Heimendinger et al. 1981). Such results would have decreased the cost per success considerably.

The second program USAID reviewed was part of a rural youth program (for 15- to 25-year-olds) aimed at increasing nutrition knowledge, production, and consumption. Activities included visits to stores, gardening projects, and discussions. The evaluation began after the project had been in effect for a year, comparing changes in participants' diets with changes in the diets of a set of controls in another community. To the surprise of the evaluators, over a third of both participants and controls showed an unfavorable change in their dietary habits over a year's time, with only a very small percentage of either group showing a favorable change.

The USAID field guide was further tested in an evaluation of two nutrition education programs in the Philippines, one of which was partially concerned with improving the dietary practices of lactating women (Jones and Munger 1978). Women were instructed in all phases of home economics through homemakers classes which met once a week for three to four hours over a year. The evaluation of impact was based on specific changes in the women's dietary habits as compared with a control group. Dietary practices were recorded prior to project implementation, after six months, and again at completion of the project. At both the six-month and one-year measurements, there was no significant increase in the number of participants who had improved diets. However, the dietary habits of a significantly higher percentage of the control group had deteriorated, indicating that the program had a positive impact in preventing an apparently normal worsening of a mother's diet during lactation. Cost data were reported for the program as a whole, of which the nutrition education component was only one part. The costs per success of the maternal nutrition educational project, were, therefore, unavailable from the published report.

The Council for Social Development (1976) compared the results of two types of health education programs for rural women in

India. The first was a functional literacy class which combined the development of literacy skills with improvements in knowledge about health and nutrition. The second program used oral instruction and demonstrations combined with a food supplement and the provision of medical services. Both classes were conducted in villages by auxiliary nurse midwives six times a week in the evening for approximately two hours. The evaluation indicated much higher participation rates in the second program; these women showed greater gains in knowledge in all areas (health, nutrition, family planning) than women in the functional literacy class. However, as might be expected, the women in the literacy program showed greater gains in literacy, although the results were not impressive.

Project Poshak in India (Gopaldas et al. 1975) contained a health and nutrition education component consisting of fortnightly visits by paraprofessionals to villages to conduct education sessions. Although the impact of the education component on women's nutritional status was not measured directly, information was collected on factors affecting participation. The authors concluded that the major reasons for nonparticipation by mothers were conflicts with work and household chores and lack of interest.

Following the national mass media health education campaign in Tanzania (for which there are no evaluation data as yet), a smaller scale participatory health education project was implemented (Stanley 1978). The program's objective was to improve women's participation in the community in identifying and solving their own health problems. Education methods included mass media presentations and small group discussions. Stanley shows community participation increased, but offers no information on the success of the programs developed by the communities in improving nutritional status.

With an aim to cure severe malnutrition among children, rehabilitation centers usually stress educating mothers about infant-feeding practices. That these centers are often successful, not only in alleviating malnutrition in the target child but in preventing it in siblings (Zeitlin and Formacion 1981) suggests that nutrition education efforts can be successful in changing women's practices, at least in regard to their children. Whether their motivation is as high to change their behaviors in regard to their own nutritional status is unknown.

Although the above evaluations are limited and in no way form a representative sample of nutrition education efforts in developing countries, a few tentative generalizations can be drawn. Increased literacy among women is an important goal. However, the use of literacy programs to improve nutrition and health will probably not be evident in the short term. More impressive results are likely to come from nutrition education programs based on demonstrations and oral instructions. Programs which can be integrated with women's work and household responsibilities will probably be more successful in reaching women than traditional classroom-oriented programs.

Most of the programs above showed a declining impact at some point after completion. This phenomenon indicates the necessity of either extending the length of the program or periodically repeating their major messages over a long period of time. Program evaluation should also take this phenomenon into consideration and not draw conclusions based on evaluations during or immediately following a program.

The occurrence in two of the above studies of a decline in nutrition knowledge and practice over time, especially among the control groups, suggests the need for further research into changes in women's nutrition practices with age, physiological status, and other factors. A project showing no clear-cut improvement in dietary behavior may still be considered successful if it arrests an otherwise normal decline.

Although the success of nutrition education programs to date has been limited, the potential benefits are clear. Often, malnutrition is the result of poor practices rather than inadequate resources. The major questions are whether to promote specific nutrition education or traditional formal education as a means of improving dietary behaviors, and how to identify the most effective ways to achieve significant long-term changes in dietary behaviors.

Price Subsidies

Subsidizing the price of certain foods is practiced by governments in developing countries, usually more for political and economic reasons than for nutritional reasons (Rogers et al. 1981; Taylor et al. 1980). However, such policies can have a nutritional impact on women. By increasing household purchasing power, price subsidies can increase the amount of food available to the household. By changing the relative prices of foods, price subsidies can affect the nutritional quality of foods available to the household. Such policies are effective in increasing household consumption only in low-income populations. Where resources are adequate and malnutrition stems from inadequate knowledge, such policies will be ineffective. Specifically, such policies cannot change the intrahousehold distribution of food and thus may not benefit women as much as other family members. Finally, price subsidies do not reach those who do not participate in the market economy, generally the poorest of the poor (Rogers et al. 1981; UN 1979b).

Evaluations of price subsidies on the basis of improvements in nutritional status have been extremely rare. Taylor et al. (1980) review a number of food subsidy programs of which only the U.S. Food Stamp Program was evaluated in terms of its impact on nutritional status (specifically, household dietary intake). Since the nutritional impact was felt to be minimal, the overall conclusion regarding the Food Stamp Program was that it acts more as an income transfer program than as a nutrition program. In the United States, the marginal propensity to consume extra food per dollar of food stamp subsidy is about 0.4 to 0.6 (Popkin et al. 1980). This means that about half the food stamp bonus is substituted for nonfood items. No studies have examined the program's effects on women's diets or nutritional status.

It has been calculated that a subsidized food ration system in Pakistan improved intake among the second lowest income group by 8.6 percent of calorie requirements and by 24 percent of protein requirements. Studies of a subsidized food program in Sri Lanka found that the subsidized ration contributed 20 percent of total household caloric intake for the lowest income group (Rogers et al. 1981). However, a study by Gavan and Chandrasekera (1979) indicates that most of the subsidized ration was substituted for open market purchases, such that the average marginal dietary increase from one pound of subsidized rice was only 0.06 pounds of rice and 0.07 pounds of cereal. Less substitution was found among the lowest income classes. These evaluations were based on per capita measures of food purchased through the subsidy program and not on actual dietary intakes. Thus, the impact specifically on the overall household diet or on women cannot be estimated.

Food price subsidy programs are often compared with income maintenance programs in which cash payments are made to households which can spend the additional income any way they desire, not necessarily on food alone. The value of the increase in food consumption, then, is likely to be less than the value of the cash received. Even in a food price subsidy program, the total increase in household food consumption is likely to be less than the value of the subsidy received because of a decrease in food purchases from other income sources. However, the increase in food consumption under a food price subsidy program is often higher than under an income maintenance program, as U.S. researchers found in comparing the Food Stamp Program with income maintenance (McDonald 1977). A similar relationship has been demonstrated in Sri Lanka, where a one dollar increase in income was found to produce an increase in the value of food consumed ranging from 22 cents in high-income groups to 58 cents in low-income groups. Receipt of one dollar's worth of subsidized food resulted in an overall increase in the value of food consumed to 84 cents (Gavan and Chandrasekera 1979).

A comparison between food price subsidies and other delivery systems with respect to their cost effectiveness in improving women's nutritional status remains to be made. With careful planning, price subsidy programs could be useful in combating malnutrition among women. Using a variation of the methodology Pinstrup-Anderson et al. (1976) developed, price elasticities of a variety of foods consumed by low-income and malnourished women could be estimated. By combining these estimations with information on the impact of increased consumption of certain foods on specific nutrient deficiencies, it is possible to identify foods which, if subsidized, would lead to a reduction in nutrient deficiencies among malnourished women. Of course, other factors also need to be considered when choosing a commodity to subsidize. The government must be able to insure supplies of the food adequate to meet the expected increase in demand. As Taylor et al. (1980) point out, in the short run, subsidy programs almost always require additional food imports. However, with appropriate input subsidies, local production can in the long run be increased to meet at least part of the additional demand.

Food Fortification

For certain specific nutrient deficiencies, food fortification is becoming a more widely practiced form of nutrition intervention (Austin et al. 1981b). Common deficiencies which appear to be amenable to correction through fortification include iodine deficiency (producing goiter), vitamin A deficiency (causing xerophthalmia), iron and folate deficiencies, and, to a lesser extent, protein deficiency. As women are vulnerable to each of these types of nutritional inadequacy, food fortification may improve their nutritional status through improvements in the quality of food consumed.

Evaluation of fortification programs has shown that, when well planned, they can be an effective and efficient means of alleviating specific nutrient deficiencies. Iodization programs have generally been effective in reducing the incidence of goiter. Iron fortification programs to reduce the prevalence of anemia have been less effective, possibly because of the poor absorption of elemental iron. Austin et al. (1981b) report on the cost effectiveness of several fortification schemes. The cost of eliminating goiter in areas of the world where it is endemic was estimated to be 20 cents per target person per year. In Guatemala, the annual cost per target person of fortifying sugar with iron was calculated to be 11 cents.

As with price subsidy programs, the effectiveness of a fortification program depends on the extent of participation by the target group in the market economy. Care must also be taken to identify foods women commonly consume.

If such foods are fortified with the deficient nutrients, a fortification program could be successful in alleviating specific nutrient deficiencies in women.

Formulated Foods

The development of formulated foods was heralded at one time as the answer to malnutrition in developing countries, but the field results of such programs have not generally borne out these high hopes (Austin et al. 1978a). Early formulated foods were highly processed and therefore quite expensive. Their use by low-income households often leads to the displacement of a larger quantity of indigenous foods and thus a possible decline in nutritional status (Popkin and Latham 1973). More recently, formulated food programs have tended toward the development of multimixes, using primarily locally available ingredients. The emphasis in the development of formulated foods has been in producing low-cost, highly nutritious weaning foods, although the products are occasionally promoted for use by the entire family.

Incaparina, a high-protein, cereal-based beverage, is one

of the oldest formulated foods, and one of the few targeted at the whole household. Although the concept has been defended (Scrimshaw 1980), the product has had only modest success in alleviating malnutrition. In a survey in Guatemala in 1965 (several years after Incaparina was introduced), 67 percent of the families interviewed knew of the product and 45 percent were consuming it. Of those consuming it, 12 percent reserved it for children and 79 percent served it to all family members. However, it is not known whether family members, especially women, consumed enough of the product to make a nutritional difference. Another study in 1968 indicated that 37 percent of families used Incaparina regularly, but there was no indication of how much women consumed (Heimendinger et al. 1981). Other studies have indicated that Incaparina is used most frequently by middle-income groups and that at current levels of production, only a small fraction of the target groups could consume it in recommended quantities.

Most successful food supplementation programs for women have used some form of formulated foods. Whether the sale of such foods in the market place would have a similar impact on women's nutritional status is unknown. To circumvent the problem of inequitable intrahousehold food distribution, careful research would have to be undertaken to identify a type of food more likely to be consumed by women than by other family members. It is not clear whether the benefits of such an approach could outweigh the costs.

HEALTH CARE PROGRAMS

Because of the complex interrelationships between health and nutrition, many health care programs can have a positive effect on the nutritional status of women. For instance, the availability of appropriate primary care services for women can improve their nutritional status by treating and curing diseases which increase nutritional needs. Improved environmental services can reduce the incidence of these nutritionally demanding infectious and parasitic diseases.

A trend has developed in recent years of incorporating nutritional services into the provision of other health care services. An American Public Health Association (APHA) survey (1977) revealed that of a nonrepresentative sample of 180 primary care projects in developing countries, 90 percent offered some nutrition services and 74 percent were actively working towards objectives in nutrition. Forty percent of the projects addressed their nutrition services to the entire community while 13 percent targeted their efforts to children and mothers together, and an additional 2 percent to mothers alone. Thus, in 55 percent of the primary health care projects surveyed, women were potential recipients of nutrition services. The rationale for this integration rests on the assumptions that:

1. The services will act synergistically and have a greater effect than the sum of the individual effects of separate programs
2. By using some of the same resources, costs of an integrated program will be less than the sum of the individual costs of separate programs
3. By providing several services at the same time and place, the time requirements of seeking care will be substantially reduced.

Evaluations of the effectiveness of integrated programs have been few, and most have concentrated on the effects of child health. The APHA report cited above states that "relatively few projects articulate goals in such fashion that it is possible to determine that they have or have not been achieved" (p. 11). Less than a dozen programs stated goals and objectives in such a manner that they could readily be evaluated. Those programs that have been evaluated have been relatively small-scale field studies with a heavy input of professional health workers, good management and surveillance, and a high level of staff motivation. Whether such results could be reproduced on a national scale is debatable.

Austin et al. (1981a) review the success of several integrated programs in reducing mortality rates. The significant decrease in infant mortality rates in all programs indicates the effectiveness of prenatal care (nutritional and medical), which suggests a possible improvement in maternal nutritional status. However, no information is included on either the short-term or long-term changes in maternal nutritional status. Gwatkin et al. (1980) review the impact of ten primary health care programs, many with a nutrition component. Again, their evaluation is based on improvements in child health and development. However, they point out that the more successful program components include maternal food supplementation and immunization against tetanus; these services are likely to improve maternal health and nutritional status, as well as child health. In terms of characteristics of successful delivery systems, they point to the use of well-trained paraprofessionals for delivery of nutrition services.

The Narangwal Nutrition Study, conducted in India between 1968 and 1973, is perhaps the most complete evaluation of the concept of integration (Kielmann et al. 1978). Several villages were provided with a variety of service combinations--either nutrition services alone, medical care services alone, a combination of nutritional and medical services, or no services (the control villages). The nutrition program included supplementation of at-risk pregnant women, as well as children. The impressive decline in perinatal mortality rates in the villages receiving the nutrition intervention over those which did not again suggests an improvement in maternal nutritional status. Unfortunately, this impact was not investigated further. Regarding the benefits of integration, the authors concluded that the effects of the two components (nutrition and medical care) were not synergistic, but that the integrated programs achieved effects similar to those of each of the separate programs with only a slight increase in expenditures. Combining the components saved 20 percent over the cost of running two separate programs; integrating nutrition, medical care, and family planning services saved 16 percent more.

Many of the programs discussed in the section on maternal supplementation also included the provision of primary health care services. However, there is rarely any information on the relative contribution to success of the different program components. Increases in dietary intakes can probably be ascribed to the supplementation program. The effects of the increased dietary intake on long-term measures of nutritional health (such as weight gain and biochemical indicators) are undoubtedly mediated by aspects of the medical care component. However, this issue has not been adequately studied in adults.

FAMILY PLANNING AND NUTRITION PROGRAMS

The nutritional problems of women associated with uncontrolled fertility and the potential nutritional problems associated with various contraceptive methods have prompted both family planning and nutrition program planners to attempt a cooperative effort. Nutrition and family planning programs are typically aimed at similar target groups which further strengthens the case for cooperation among these sectors. Their cooperation also makes use of scarce country resources, both financial and staff. Family planning workers have been persuaded of the need for nutritional counseling for their clients by the suggestion that some of the side-effects of contraceptive usage, such as depression and skin rashes among orals users and excess bleeding of IUD users, might be mitigated through dietary modifications (Adams et al. 1973; Ahmed et al. 1975; Guillebaud et al. 1976). Some family planners have also suggested that providing a service such as nutrition counseling can draw clients to family planning participation since it can alleviate some of the potential hesitation about using family planning services (Johnson and Meyer 1977). The high frequency of client contact commonly available through nutrition programs has also been suggested as potentially valuable to family planning through repeated reinforcement of the family-planning messages as well as contraceptive method acceptor follow-up which may importantly reduce drop-out rates (Austin 1981). Nutrition planners, on the other hand, have obvious interest in the promotion of breast-feeding and of nutritional well-being for women as well as for all household members. We have reviewed the intimate relationship of family planning to these concerns elsewhere. Additionally, Austin notes that beyond the effectiveness and efficiency of service provision aspects, the integration of family planning and nutrition has other benefits: population programming, although highly justifiable in economic terms, may nonetheless be saddled with substantial political obstacles while nutrition programming may often be considered a political asset but is more difficult to justify economically even under a "human capital" development objective. Austin suggests that an integrated program package might have more opportunity for government support, in that case, than either program alone.

Although literature touting the rationale for integrating these services is substantial, little information is available on the impact of such integrated programs. Not only are studies needed on the effects on the nutritional status of women participants, but also on the degree of acceptance of both services among the target populations and administrative solutions to the problems of providing integrated services.

Although nutrition and family planning appear well-suited for cooperation, difficulties in implementing such programming are many. In those countries where nutrition and family planning services are either scanty or not well organized, the possibilities are enhanced for integrated services through implementation of a new or more widespread distribution of these services. In those countries where nutrition or family planning services are numerous and well-organized, the difficulties associated with forging agreements among entrenched bureaucracies are immense.

Criteria for obtaining funding for nutrition and family planning programs may require performance standards based on reductions in malnutrition and acceptance and continued use of some contraceptive method. Integrated programming may be more loosely structured around cooperation for referrals and general information about respective programs. Integrated programs which might give credit to workers for referrals or information alone would not only be difficult to monitor and evaluate but also to defend in tight budget situations. In such cases, territorial concerns and the ability to monitor the quantity and quality of services and outcomes may be important determinants of the success and longevity of the integrated programs.

Further complications include reimbursement of ministries and their field workers or private groups for integrated work where multiple agencies are involved in nutrition and family planning work. There may also be problems with decisions about the extent to which field workers will be trained respectively to do nutrition or family planning work, as well as setting target output expectations for that work. In the case of training and output expectations, resistance may be encountered in both groups to allowing the others to take over some of their "professional" tasks. A Ford Foundation field exploration of integrated health programs found difficulties in program implementation including

> bureaucratic rigidities, both on the part of donors and government agencies, the limitations of sectoral agencies for adequate coverage and integration of services, feuds and schism between government agencies, limited absorptive

capacity, top-down initiation and management of projects, the "medicalized" approach and lip service to research and evaluation. (Simmons 1981, 22)

Additional constraints included "management incapacity, cost factors, and the questionable capacity of field workers to deliver a package of services" (p. 12).

Besides the health sector, other areas have provided opportunities for nutrition and family planning cooperation. Agricultural extension is an important example. USAID has provided several years of support for family planning education through home economist services via a contract with the American Home Economics Association's international projects office. Resource materials, training, and consultations have been made available to various developing countries with home economist services. In the Philippines, the Bureau of Agricultural Extension has, since the early 1970s, been actively training its home management technicians in family planning and directing them to promote family planning practice among their clients. These technicians typically provide education to women in various home economics areas including a strong emphasis on practical aspects of foods and nutrition for the family.

Austin et al. (1981a) describe national, regional, and community level readiness for the ideal country situation for implementing integrated programming. It is clear, however, that integrated programming is proceeding without the benefit of such an approach, given the political and bureaucratic complexities of implementing such ideas.

Program types suggested for the integration of nutrition and family planning services range from informal agreements for referrals between nutrition and family planning services to independent units which provide a full range of services, including community health workers who provide both services (Johnson and Meyer 1977). Such integrated full service programs have typically existed within units providing primary health care, sometimes for the community at large and more often for mothers and children. The Narangwal Project (Kielmann et al. 1978) typifies the community program, and the Taylor-Berelson projects (Lapham and Van Wie 1976) in Kenya, the Philippines, Indonesia, and Turkey is an example of the maternal and child health approach.

The bottom line to this discussion, however, is unknown. Even if nutrition-family planning services could be implemented, it is not possible to state with precision what the impact would be on women's nutrition status. There is a potentially strong positive effect on women's nutritional status through family planning practice. Evaluations of existing programs will be needed to substantiate this idea, however.

DEVELOPMENT PROGRAMS

Development programs can have a significant impact on thenutritional status of all segments of a population, including women. It is generally believed that by increasing income, most development programs will have a positive impact on women's nutritional status. However, the consequences of development are complex, and, as a number of authors point out (Boserup 1970; Javillonar et al. 1979; Whyte and White 1978), do not always result in improvements in the lives of women. The relative positive and negative impacts of development directly on women's nutritional status have not been studied, but the impact of development programs on many of the determinants of women's nutritional status have been suggested or documented by a few authors. In this section, we review some of the mechanisms by which development may affect the nutritional status of women. Since there appears to be a spectrum of unfortunate consequences for women in the processes of development, this review may appear to be largely negative. Women have only recently begun to be considered as a separate entity in planning development projects and the impacts of these "women in development" programs have not yet been evaluated.

Development programs often are designed to improve the income of the target population. However, improving household income may not improve the nutritional status of women. Development specialists are becoming increasingly aware of the different functions of men's and women's income. In many societies, women's income is more likely to be used to provide basic necessities while men's income may be used for luxuries or for capital investments (Engle 1980; Guyer 1980; Palmer 1980). Thus, development programs which emphasize an increase in income-producing activities men typically engage in (e.g., cash cropping) may not improve the nutritional status of women and children as much as programs which increase women's income-generating possibilities. Even if an increase in household income did result in an increase in household food availability, the prevailing patterns of intrahousehold food distribution may prevent any significant positive effect on the nutritional status of women. Dixon (1980) mentions another interesting mechanism by which increased household income may actually produce a decline in women's nutritional status. In societies practicing purdah, as a low-income family improves its income and status, it is more likely that the women will withdraw from society and may have a higher prevalence of vitamin D deficiency (from lack of exposure to sunlight) and a higher prevalence of obesity (from inactivity).

Another common objective of development programs is to increase agricultural productivity. On the surface, it would appear that such programs would be likely to have a positive impact on the nutritional status of women, but this may not be the case. Such programs frequently emphasize the growing of cash crops, which may be grown on the prime agricultural land, forcing subsistence crops to poorer land, resulting in lower yields (World Bank 1979). Cash cropping may also divert labor from subsistence crop growing, resulting in a decrease in food production. Dixon (1980) discusses such a consequence of a rice irrigation scheme in Kenya. The project increased the amount of time women spent in the rice fields and decreased the amount of time they spent on garden plots. Rice production and income increased but nutritional status declined.

Development projects also have a significant impact on women's time. Recent studies have shown that, in a number of cases, development programs have increased the amount of time women spend at work relative to men (Birdsall and McGreevey 1983; Palmer 1979). This means they may have less time available for the production and preparation of food and their nutritional status, as well as that of other family members, may suffer as a consequence. In addition to increased time demands, development programs may also increase women's levels of physical activity (ADC 1975; Palmer 1980), which increases their nutritional needs. If these increased needs are not met by increased intake, nutritional status may decline. Increased work loads for adult women often imply increased work loads for young girls, either as household substitutes or as additional income generators (Evenson et al. 1979). This may result in lower educational levels for girls which, to the extent that education fosters improvement in nutritional status, may have a negative impact on their future nutritional status (Palmer 1980).

It is often assumed, based on gross comparisons of societies in different stages of development, that the relationship between development and fertility is inverse--that improvements in income brought about by development lessens the demand for a large family. Fertility declines would have a positive impact on women's nutritional status by reducing the nutritional demands of repeated pregnancies and periods of lactation. However, as Palmer (1980) points out, an agricultural development policy based on expanding the use of family labor may have a positive impact on fertility. The more children there are, the more the family can produce.

A final corollary of development that needs to be considered in light of its impact on women's nutritional status is the phenomenon of the female-headed household. Buvinić and Youssef (1978) discuss the growing percentage of women household heads in developing countries. Many of the reasons for this trend are directly related to the development process. For instance, migration of men from rural to urban areas in search of employment often leaves women as de facto household heads. Because a woman heads a household does not automatically imply that its members are at increased nutritional risk. However, female-headed households are more likely to incorporate many of the characteristics linked with poor nutritional status, such as low income, lower educational levels of the head, less time available for food production and preparation, and lower social status. Thus, women who head households may be more likely to be malnourished than their counterparts in male-headed households.

Palmer (1979) reports a case study of some potentially negative consequences of inappropriately planned development. The study was an amalgam of two development projects, both of which sought to increase income. One project involved an irrigation scheme and reform of land ownership, giving land for both cash crops (rice) and subsistence crops to each household. The other project involved increasing the catch of local fishermen by supplying them with power boats and arranging for commercial processing and sale of the fish. In the first project, women household heads initially suffered because land was apportioned only to households with a male head. Additionally, only males were allowed membership in the Farmer's Association, the local extension service. Thus the women did not receive extension aid for the growing of subsistence crops. Women in the fishing village no longer had access to the surplus catch and thus could not as readily serve fish to the families. Both their families' and their own nutritional status may have declined as a result, although no data are given. Also, because the men were now engaged full-time in fishing, women had to work both the rice fields and the subsistence fields, increasing their time and energy demands and possibly decreasing the amount of time available for food preparation. Because of their increased time demands, the women did not have time to implement much of the nutritional advice being offered by the newly organized health service. Although it is not clear that the overall effect of the projects was negative, it is possible they were detrimental to the nutritional status of some groups of women.

One of the most promising trends in development theory and practice in terms of a potential positive impact on women's nutritional status is the recent concern with "appropriate technologies" (Tinker 1979). An example of the application of such an idea is the promotion of hand-operated rather than machine-operated grain mills. Whereas hand-driven equipment is likely to be used by women, high level technological devices, such as machine-driven mills, are often appropriated by men, thus depriving women of a traditional source of income and status. Such small-scale technologies lessen the burden on women's time and may, at the same time, increase their income, both of which may positively affect their nutritional status. Areas where the concept of appropriate technology may have a significant impact on women's nutritional status include improving food processing and storage capabilities, improving agricultural tools, developing less energy intensive cooking methods and materials (such as solar cookers), and improving water storage and waste disposal.

Chapter 7
Policy Implications

Based on the information reviewed here, it is apparent that women in developing countries, because of their unique biological, social, and economic statuses, are at considerable risk of being malnourished. If women are considered a risk group strictly on the basis of their reproductive role (a position taken by many health professionals and program planners), then the recognition of their nutritional vulnerability caused by their other roles only adds to an already significant level of risk. And, because of their many functions in society, the consequences of poor nutritional status among women affects not only future generations of children, but current progress toward economic and social development goals. The relative risk of nonpregnant, nonlactating women versus other target groups (infants, children, pregnant and lactating women, men) varies by locality. Thus, we cannot suggest that scarce monies be unilaterally redirected from programs for children to programs for women. However, we can suggest that the risk of women be realistically evaluated in formulating policies and programs, and that specific programs involving women be based on a careful consideration of women's economic, sociocultural, and health situations.

The following paragraphs will review how some of the information discussed above on the determinants of women's nutritional status could be incorporated into the design of more successful programs and policies. In addition, major areas where further research is needed will be identified.

OVERVIEW

Physiological Status

Frequently throughout this review we have noted that pregnancy and lactation have been a major focus in both nutrition research and nutrition intervention programs in developing countries. However, interest has generally been on the impact on infant health, with maternal nutritional status as an intermediate factor. With such programs already in place in many areas of the world, it should be relatively easy to collect information on the impact of pregnancy and lactation on maternal nutritional status, as well as data on the effectiveness of various intervention schemes in improving maternal nutrition. Such information is badly needed for the effective design of programs to improve women's nutritional health.

Most mothers want healthy children. Thus the motivation of women to seek medical and nutritional care during pregnancy and lactation may be higher than during nonpregnant, nonlactating periods (Akin et al. 1981). Programs to improve women's long-term nutritional status could capitalize on this motivation by initially attracting pregnant and lactating women, but continuing to provide services beyond the immediate childbearing period.

The effects of the use of hormonal contraceptives on nutritional status are not yet clear enough to make specific policy recommendations. Further research is needed on the functional effects of altered blood levels of certain nutrients among users of oral contraceptives as well as on the effects of supplementation. Women using intrauterine devices should be considered a high-risk group nutritionally, in view of the increased risks of anemia associated with heavy blood loss. The prevalence of infectious and parasitic diseases (particularly hookworm, malaria, and schistosomiasis) among women in developing countries and their possible impact on nutritional status indicates the need for giving special nutritional attention to women afflicted with these diseases. Treatment of the disease should include treatment of any underlying nutritional problems. Women suffering from these diseases should be carefully considered for inclusion in food supplementation programs. In particular, pregnant women with malaria could be targeted for protein-calorie supplementation, in addition to what their pregnancy requires, in order to compensate for the increased calorie and protein losses brought about by the disease. Further research needs to be conducted on the extent of various diseases among women, and their functional effects; for example, the effects of malaria on lactation performance needs clarification.

Income and Assets

It is generally believed that as income increases, nutritional status improves. While this relationship may be clear for total household food consumption or for the nutritional status of children, it is not clear what the effect of income is on women's nutritional status. One factor modifying the usual income-diet relationship may be the prevailing patterns of intrahousehold food distribution. Another factor concerns the access women have to an increase in household income. Income accruing to women rather than men may be more likely to be spent on food. Both of these factors need to be carefully considered within any culture before any assumptions can be made on the impact of women's nutritional status of income-generating programs.

Time and Work

Designers of any program targeted to women in developing countries must take into consideration the well-documented fact that women face heavy constraints on their time. Any program which puts further demands on women's time is likely to have limited success, especially in terms of reaching the neediest women who are often those with the least free time available. This situation suggests delivering services at or near women's work locations. A good example of such a program is a nutrition education program which involved playing nutrition-related tape recordings while women carried on their daily washing (Colle and Fernandez de Colle 1978). Nutrition supplementation programs could also be operated at the work place. At the very least, programs should dispense services at times of the day, week, and year at which the target women are likely to be relatively free of other responsibilities, and should keep the demands on women's time to a minimum.

Reducing the overall demands on women's time may improve their nutritional status but this issue requires more study. While it is clear that introducing appropriate labor-saving technology may indeed reduce women's time constraints, it is not clear that women will spend that extra time on home food production and preparation. However, if such labor-savings techniques result in a substantial reduction in women's energy expenditures, some improvement in their nutritional status can be expected.

Household Size and Structure

Based on the current state of knowledge, large household size is felt to be detrimental to a woman's nutritional health. The economic gains achieved by having an increased number of family workers in a large family appear to be offset by the nutritional costs of repeated pregnancies and periods of lactation as well as the drain on household resources by these extra persons. Therefore, family-planning programs should continue to be emphasized and, if successful, can be expected to have a long-term positive impact on women's nutritional status.

The increasing prevalence in developing countries of households headed by women will need to receive more consideration from nutrition planners. Female household heads are generally subject to even heavier income, time and social constraints than women in male-headed households. For the purposes of nutrition planning, such women should be considered a special risk group with extra efforts needed to provide them with appropriate services.

Intrahousehold Issues

The question of intrahousehold distribution of food is crucial to the success of most forms of nutrition intervention. Providing food to a household does not guarantee that women will receive an increased share. That women eat last and least in most cultures is a generally accepted notion, although documentation is scarce. In order to improve a woman's share of available food resources, it is important to know what factors determine the current patterns of distribution. It has been suggested that improving women's economic status will improve the equity of intrahousehold food distribution, but this hypothesis is as yet untested. For the purposes of current program planning, it is necessary to know to what extent, among the target population, women suffer from inequitable distribution. If it is significant, then means of circumventing the problem need to be considered. In some cases it is not the wife who necessarily prepares food or makes the decisions regarding food use and distribution. Instead, it may be a husband, mother-in-law, or other adult family member. Alternatives to the allocation program, then, include on-site feeding rather than take-home programs, identifying an appropriate "women's food," and increasing its availability or fortifying it, or increasing the quantity of food available to the entire household to such an extent that some of the extra will be left over for the women.

Seasonal Variations

The effects of seasonal fluctuations in food consumption, time, income, and disease prevalence of women have been grossly overlooked by program planners. Seasonality affects not only women's nutritional needs (because of higher work loads and increased disease prevalence during peak agricultural periods) and their resources for meeting those needs (related to reduced food and income resources and increased food prices during the preharvest season), but also affects the ability of programs to reach women physically (because of lack of transportation during rainy seasons and lack of women's time). Development programs can be implemented which will smooth out some of these seasonal fluctuations. Improving food storage facilities may decrease wastage and ensure the availability of food during the usual periods of food shortage. Irrigation projects allow for staggered crop planting and harvesting which eliminates some of the fluctuation in women's time inputs to agricultural tasks, as well as equalizing the year-round availability of food. Specific nutrition intervention programs need to be designed with enough flexibility to incorporate changes in needs during various seasons. For instance, supplementation programs may need to increase the level of supplementation during the preharvest season, or may need to deliver food directly to women in the fields during planting and harvesting periods. Health and nutrition programs also need to be aware of the seasonal fluctuations in the prevalence of nutritionally damaging diseases and plan programs accordingly.

Urban Residence

The relative nutritional status of urban versus rural women is an issue not clear enough yet to warrant specific program and policy recommendations. Although much anecdotal information exists, very little good research has been done on the specific problems of urban women, or in determining the most effective delivery systems for providing them with nutritional services. Given the apparent wider availability of foodstuffs and services in the urban areas of some countries, addressing nutritional problems in the cities may involve augmenting income to make different nutrients or resources available and providing education and training in more efficient health and nutrition practices.

Education and Information

Program planners designing nutrition intervention strategies for women need awareness of the general level of education and literacy among women in the region. Considering the general low literacy levels among poor women, nutrition education programs should rely on demonstrations and oral instruction. Further research needs to be conducted on the impact of general education versus nutrition education on women's nutritional status. Education methods which maintain improvements in dietary practices over time need further delineation. Specific attention should also be given to assessing changes in the availability and use of traditional dietary items and to revising existing concepts of food use and disease causation where necessary.

Cultural Preferences

The constraints imposed on women's nutritional status by cultural taboos need much further research. Although examples of such taboos abound in the literature, it is not clear to what extent they are actually practiced and whether they are amenable to change. Until such information is available, planners need to be aware of local taboos and design intervention strategies around them. Changes in household nutrition cannot be sustained without accounting for the social networks which affect the behavior and opinions of individual household members. It may be advantageous to target influential households or women in a community when implementing an intervention program.

Targeting

A final program-related issue concerns the question of targeting. As mentioned in the section on food supplementation programs, targeting involves both costs and savings. When considering expanding the scope of current nutrition intervention efforts to include all women at risk, targeting becomes a necessity. Targets usually are set at two levels, the community and the individual or household. Community targets are often based on socioeconomic indicators, such as per capita income or land ownership (Popkin 1981). As discussed in the section on income, the situation of women is usually not reported in official statistics. Therefore, any targeting of nutrition programs based solely on such data may overlook communities with a significant number of women at risk. Efforts should be made to assess specifically the status of women rather than their households when designating areas to receive nutrition programs.

Relatively simple individual or household eligibility criteria can probably be implemented in a cost-effective manner by most developing countries. However, a few cautions are in order. Targets based on biological characteristics such as anthropometric measurements or the presence of debilitating diseases require the contribution of trained health workers, but have the advantage of possibly inducing greater use of health facilities. Targeting based on income must overcome the difficulties involved in equating subsistence activities with income-generating activities. Providing benefits on the basis of family structure characteristics (such as female head or number of children) may actually promote socially undesirable situations. It is probably more reasonable to consider such women as eligible only if they meet other income or biologic criteria, but they may require a different type or level of service. It is clear that targeting criteria need to be tailored to local conditions.

CONCLUSION

The data on women's nutrition, nutritional determinants, and intervention programs support very strongly the need for comprehensive approaches to development planning. The various factors influencing women's nutrition are interactive in their effects, and programs which attempt to address women's nutritional status must reflect this. Resources and income, or the availability of products and facilities in themselves, do not appear adequate to sustain the improvement in family nutrition or women's health. Without training and education in the appropriate means of selecting and preparing foods and supplements, for example, many programs have been marked for failure. On the other hand, information and awareness alone will not allow women or their households to modify their habits. One of the most important but overlooked factors in the change of nutritional behavior is the cultural impact of others (e.g., community leaders, information networks) in defining what is the acceptable and preferred behavior.

Without a comprehensive assessment of and attention to resource needs, information, and training, as well as social acceptability, the nutritional differences between poor and wealthy women and their families will continue to multiply. Early ethnographic commentators like Richards (1939) noted that differences in food consumption between rich and poor members of the societies they studied (as yet barely affected by industrial urbanization) occurred mostly in terms of supply and quantity. Today qualitative differences in diet and nutrition reflect the exacerbation of these differences over time and as a result of industrial development. Women's unique dietary needs and roles in household nutrition and family well-being require serious attention if their nutritional status is to be significantly improved.

Notes

1.   We use the following definitions: *neonatal mortality* = number of deaths during the first 28 days of life per 1,000 live births; *perinatal mortality* = number of deaths from the 28th week of gestation to the 7th day of life per 1,000 live births; *infant mortality* = number of deaths during the first year of life per 1,000 live births..

2.   We address only the nutritional impacts on biological components of fertility. A large body of literature has explored the psychosocial connection between the effects of improved nutritional status on lowering infant and child mortality rates, and subsequent changes in fertility behavior. The major decision-making strategies proposed to account for fertility responses to infant and child mortality are outside the scope of this review. See Rutherford 1975; Schultz 1976; Wray 1978; and Zeitlin et al. 1983.

Appendix A

CONTRIBUTORS OF MATERIALS AND IDEAS

Carol Adelman, U.S. Agency for International Development, Washington, DC

Dr. H. Hekmat Aly, U.S. Agency for International Development, Cairo, Egypt

Samir Basta, International Bank for Reconstruction and Development, Washington, DC

Patricia Blair, Equity Policy Center, Washington, DC

Boston Women's Health Collective, Boston, MA

Elena Brineman, U.S. Agency for International Development, Washington, DC

Art Braunstein, U.S. Agency for International Development, Washington, DC

Thierry Brun, Groupe de Recherche Appliquée, Interdisciplinaire sur la Nutrition et le Santé, Paris, France

Mayra Buvinic, International Center for Research on Women, Washington, DC

Adolfo Chávez, Institute of Nutrition, Mexico City

Olfat Darwish, School of Public Health, Alexandria, Egypt

V. Reggie Edgerton, University of California, Los Angeles

Gayle Gibbons, American Public Health Association, Washington, DC

Diane Hedgecock, National Council for International Health, Washington, DC

Darwin Karyadi, Nutrition Research Institute, Bogor, Indonesia

Emily Leonard, U.S. Agency for International Development, Cairo, Egypt

Joanne Leslie, International Bank for Reconstruction and Development, Washington, DC

Maureen Lewis, U.S. Agency for International Development, Washington, DC

Maternal and Child Health Division, World Health Organization, Geneva, Switzerland

Patricia McClure, New Transcentury Foundation, Washington, DC

Judy McGuire, Food and Nutrition Service, U.S. Department of Agriculture, Washington, DC

Nadamuni Naidu, National Institute of Nutrition, Hyderabad, India
Deborah Purcell, U.S. Agency for International Development,
    Washington, DC
David Rush, Columbia University, New York, NY
Dr. Amin Said, U.S. Agency for International Development, Cairo, Egypt
Tina Sanghvi, U.S. Agency for International Development, Washington, DC
Gloria Scott, International Bank for Reconstruction and Development,
    Washington, DC
Ozzie G. Simmons, Ford Foundation, New York City
Dinesh Sinha, Pan American Health Organization, Washington, DC
L. J. Teply, United Nations International Children's Emergency Fund,
    New York City
Benhamin Torun, Institute of Nutrition of Central America and Panama,
    Guatemala City
Carole Waslien, League for International Food Education, Washington, DC

Appendix B

Table 1. Sex Differences in Life Expectancy in Years in Selected Countries

Country & region	Year	Life expectancy at birth		Probability of survival from 15-45 years		Sex Ratios	
						In life expectancy	In survival rate
		M (1)	F (2)	M (3)	F (4)	(2) ÷ (1)	(4) ÷ (3)
AFRICA							
Egypt	1960	51.6	53.8	0.89	0.93	1.04	1.04
Liberia	1971	45.8	44.0	0.75	0.84	0.96	1.12
Mauritius	1961-63	58.7	61.9	0.91	0.89	1.05	0.98
Nigeria	1965-66	37.2	36.7	0.76	0.73	0.99	0.96
AMERICAS							
USA	1974	67.4	75.1	0.92	0.96	1.11	1.04
Canada	1970-72	69.3	76.4	0.94	0.97	1.10	1.03
Argentina	1970-75	65.1	71.4	0.87	0.89	1.10	1.02
Brazil	1960-70	57.6	61.1	0.87	0.89	1.06	1.02
Chile	1969-70	60.5	66.0	0.88	0.93	1.09	1.06
Colombia	1970-75	59.2	62.7	0.88	0.89	1.06	1.01
Jamaica	1959-61	62.7	66.6	0.91	0.92	1.06	1.01
ASIA							
Burma	1970-75	48.5	51.5	0.74	0.67	1.06	0.90
Hong Kong	1971	67.4	75.0	0.93	0.96	1.11	1.07
India	1951-60	41.0	40.6	0.70	0.63	0.99	0.90
Japan	1974	71.2	76.3	0.93	0.96	1.07	1.03
Jordan	1959-63	52.6	52.0	0.81	0.81	0.99	1.00
Khmer Republic	1958-59	44.2	43.3	0.74	0.69	0.98	0.93
Malaysia: Sabah	1970	48.8	45.4	0.87	0.77	0.93	0.89
Sarawak	1970	51.2	52.7	0.88	0.82	1.03	0.93
West M.	1970	63.4	68.0	0.91	0.93	1.07	1.02
Pakistan	1962	53.7	48.8	0.87	0.77	0.91	0.89
Philippines	1970-75	56.9	60.0	0.80	0.81	1.05	1.01
Sri Lanka	1967	64.8	66.9	0.91	0.92	1.03	1.01
Thailand	1960	53.6	58.7	0.71	0.75	1.10	1.06
Korea	1970	63.0	67.0	0.92	0.94	1.06	1.02

Source: WHO 1980c

Table 2. Death Rates from Nutrition-Related Diseases in Several Developing Countries as Compared with the U.S.

Disease	Guatamala (1976) F	Guatamala (1976) M	Nicaragua (1977) F	Nicaragua (1977) M	Iran (1978) F	Iran (1978) M	Egypt (1975) F	Egypt (1975) M	Philippines (1976) F	Philippines (1976) M	USA (1977) F	USA (1977) M
Infective & Parasitic												
ages 25-34							12.3	23.3	52.5	78.4	3.5	1.7
35-44							15.2	27.4	102.7	162.1	2.5	3.5
Total	392.0	403.4	101.8	130.9							6.9	8.8
	(30.5)	(29.4)	(21.9)	(21.2)	(12.6)	(10.9)						
Diabetes Mellitus												
ages 25-34							1.7	2.9	0.2	0.4	1.3	1.7
35-44							3.8	5.3	1.1	1.9	3.3	4.2
Total	5.4	3.9	5.3	4.2			6.6	7.0	3.0	2.8	17.4	12.9
	(0.4)	(0.3)	(1.2)	(0.7)	(0.3)	(0.2)						
Hypertensive Disease												
ages 25-34							2.3	3.4	3.2	4.2	0.3	0.5
35-44							9.9	9.2	9.5	16.3	1.2	1.7
Total	4.8	3.6	1.9	1.5			28.1	29.8	16.4	21.9	8.1	6.8
	(0.4)	(0.3)	(0.4)	(0.2)	(1.0)	(0.8)						
Ischemic Heart Disease												
ages 25-34							1.6	4.1	4.8	11.8	1.7	6.8
35-44							5.0	16.6	14.3	32.6	14.6	63.5
Total	4.3	4.9	8.6	9.0			8.4	23.3	25.9	37.2	255.1	337.2
	(0.3)	(0.4)	(1.8)	(1.4)	(2.3)	(2.4)						
Cerebro-Vascular Disease												
ages 25-34							1.5	3.7	2.0	4.9	2.9	3.2
35-44							3.4	5.6	7.1	12.4	10.1	10.1
Total	8.8	8.4	19.3	18.9			6.7	9.4	9.9	13.0	94.1	73.5
	(0.7)	(0.6)	(4.1)	(3.0)	(1.4)	(1.1)						
Pregnancy Complications												
ages 25-34							14.5		20.7		1.1	
35-44							14.9		29.9		0.5	
Total	12.5		7.1									
	(1.0)		(1.5)		(0.4)							

Note: Rates are per 100,000 population; numbers in parentheses are proportion of total deaths from the cause stated.

Source: WHO 1980c

Table 3. Numbers and Estimated Percentage of Women Aged 15 to 49 with Hemoglobin Concentrations below WHO Norm, by Continent

Location	Pregnant Women		Nonpregnant Women		All Women	
	N	%	N	%	N	%
Developing countries in:						
Africa	15.1	63	77.1	40	92.2	40
America	9.6	30	65.0	15	74.6	17
Asia (excluding China)	43.2	65	253.2	57	296.4	58
Oceania	0.1	58	0.9	71	1.0	70
Total	68.0	60	396.2	47	464.2	49

Notes: Number in millions of women.

WHO standards for deficient hemoglobin concentrations: Adult females, nonpregnant, < 120g/l; pregnant, < 110 g/l

Source: WHO 1979

Table 4. Summary of Studies on Prevalence of Hypertension

Location	Sample	Measure	F	M	Total
Indonesia[1]	Clinic patients 30-39 yrs. (13F, 16M)	$\overline{X}$ diastolic	108.0	108.0	
	40-49 yrs. (28F, 29M)	$\overline{X}$ diastolic % > 160 mm	115.0 7.2%	110.6 3.4%	
Indonesia[2]	Healthy patients 20-29 yrs. (56F, 26M)	$\overline{X}$ % > 150 mm	115.3/71.8	110.7/66.7	0%
	30-39 yrs. (86F, 35M)	$\overline{X}$ % > 150 mm	123.8/74.4	112.5/69.0	3.3%
	40-44 yrs. (N unknown) 40-49 yrs. (77F, 65M)	$\overline{X}$ % > 150 mm	128.0/78.4 9.7%	113.0/69.2 3.8%	6.3%
Polynesia[3]	All adults on island of Pukapuka (179F, 188M)	% > 159/94 in those > age 40	7	3	
	Urban Polynesians in Rarotonga (212F, 243M)		47	28	
	Europeans in rural New Zealand (224F, 202M)		48	27	
Solomon Islands[4]	"More accul- turated" tribes (265F, 245M)	% > 140/90	3.8	4.5	
	"Less accul- turated" tribes (311F, 335M)		0.3	0.5	

Sources: (1) Shirai & Matsuo 1967; (2) Matsuo 1967; (3) Prior & Evans 1969;
(4) Page et al. 1974

Table 5. Summary of Studies on Prevalence of Diabetes Mellitus in Developing
Countries

Location	Sample	Measure	F	M	Total
ASIA					
E. Pakistan[1] (N = 513)	"Crudely representative" of all age 34; sex adjusted	% diabetic (blood glucose > 140 mg/100 ml 2 hrs after load)	2.8	1.2	1.5
India[2]	Unrepresentative 17-village screening: 20-50 yrs (671F, 885M)	% w/ glycosuria	1.2	2.5 no significant difference	1.8
Malaya[1] **(N=566)**	"Crudely representative" of all age 34; sex adjusted	% diabetic (blood glucose > 140 mg/100 ml 2 hrs after load)	2.1	4.5	3.5
Papua, New Guinea[3]	Urban: 18-34 yrs (23F, 79M)	% w/ diabetes (plasma glucose > 11.0 mmol/l 2 hrs after load	21.7	11.4	
	35-54 yrs (20F,58M)		25.0	17.2	
	Rural: 18-34 yrs (31F, 9M)		0	0	
	35-54 yrs (22F, 23M)		0	4.3	
Polynesia[4]	N unknown:	% w/ diabetes			
	Cook Island rural		1.6	0.4	
	urban		4.3	5.5	
	Tokelau Is. rural		5.9	1.9	
	urban		7.3	5.0	
	W. Samoa rural		6.2	2.8	
	urban		12.2	12.8	
LATIN AMERICA					
Costa Rica[5] (266F, 180M)	"Crudely representative"; sex adjusted	% diabetic (whole blood glucose > 149 mg/100 ml 2 hrs after glucose load)	7.5	3.3	5.4
El Salvador[5] (168F, 7M)			4.2	2.1	3.2
Guatemala[5] (294F, 204M)			5.4	2.9	4.2
Honduras[5] (208F, 134M)			6.7	1.5	4.1

Table 5. continued

Location	Sample	Measure	F	M	Total
Jamaica[6]	Rural: 77% response	% diabetic (plasma glucose > 180 ml/dl 1 hr after glucose load or positive 3-hr glucose tolerance test)			
	25-34 yrs (75F, 55M)		0	1.8	
	35-44 yrs (97F, 63M)		5.2	4.8	
	45-54 yrs (74F, 69M)		13.3	14.5	
	55-64 yrs (53F, 47M)		17.0	10.6	
Nicaragua[1] (259F, 130M)	"Crudely representative"; sex adjusted	% diabetic (whole blood glucose > 149 mg/100 ml 2 hrs after glucose load)	7.7	2.3	5.0
Panama[2] (200F, 145M)			5.0	0.0	2.5
Uruguay[5] (N = 484)	"Crudely representative of all age 34	% diabetic (blood glucose > 140 mg/100 ml 2 hrs after load)	6.9	6.8	6.9
Venezuela[5] (N = 480)			9.4	4.5	7.3

Sources: (1) West & Kalbfleisch 1966; (2) Rao et al. 1972; (3) Martin et al. 1980; (4) Zimmet 1979; (5) West & Kalbfleisch 1970; (6) Florey et al. 1972

Table 6. Deaths from Ischemic Heart Disease in Several Countries

Location	Sample	Measure	F	M
Chile	N unknown	Mortality/	86.3	117.8
Columbia		100,000 from ischemic heart	49.4	63.4
El Salvador		disease	8.0	13.9
Mexico			27.4	38.1
Panama			75.4	45.2
USA			157.4	317.7

Source: Soukupová & Průšová, 1970

Table 7. Evaluation of Nutrition Assessment Methodologies

Method	Criteria			
	Accuracy	Cost	Skill	Time
Anthropometry	high	medium	low	low
Clinical	medium	medium	high	high
Biochemical	high	high	high	medium
Dietary	medium	medium	medium	low-medium

Source: Adapted from Austin 1978

Table 8. Evaluation of Indicators of Nutritional Status

Indicator	Uses	Advantages	Limitations
Weight/ height	Measure body fullness or thinness; assess over-weight & acute malnutrition	High accuracy if done carefully; best available energy-protein malnutrition measure	Cumbersome equipment for mobile study; does not indicate malnutrition duration
Arm circumference	Measure muscle mass or protein reserves	Portable, cheap equipment; useful in assessing severe vs. mild malnutrition	Cannot be used alone as nutritional status indicator; insensitive to recent nutritional status changes; insufficient inter- and intraexaminer repeatability; needs large sample for validity due to large standard error of measurement & narrow data distribution must be used in combination with triceps fatfold measurement to assess fat & protein reserves separately
Pregnancy weight gain	Estimate fetal growth; predict infant birth weight	Simple, fast; minimal equipment	Women must visit prenatal services; frequent lack of prepregnancy weight; difficulty in dating last menstrual period; uncertainty if weight gain reflects fluid retention, excessive fat accumulation, other tissue related to products of conception vs. fetal growth; equipment may be cumbersome
Skinfold thickness	Evaluate total body fat (subcutaneous fat correlates w/ fat in body cavities); used primarily to assess obesity	Minimal, portable equipment	Low inter- and intraexaminer repeatability; problem in site selection--triceps fatfold most commonly used; accessibility of part to be measured; variability in skinfold thickness over measurement area; the fatter the subject the less reliable the measurement; expensive equipment
Hemoglobin	Determine prevalence of nutritional anemia; measure hemoglobin concentration in blood	Fingerprick sample only; needs no refrigeration; unaffected by recent meal; simple; fast; inexpensive; reliable	Does not detect short-term iron deficiency

continued

Table 8 continued

Indicator	Uses	Advantages	Limitations
Hematocrit	Determine prevalence of nutritional anemia; assess volume of packed red corpuscles in blood	More suitable for field studies than hemoglobin; otherwise identical advantages	Does not detect short-term iron deficiency
24-hour dietary recall	Assess individual nutrient intake in past 24 hrs; obtain average nutrient intakes of groups to determine dietary inadequacies in comparison to other groups or recommended intakes	Provides information on dietary habits; low respondent burden	May not reflect usual intake; accuracy partly depends on subject's memory, cooperation, & ability to quantitate food intake; interview bias; subjects may withhold or alter information; high cost relative to data obtained
Food record	Assess nutrient intake from records made at time of consumption by weighing, household measures	Provides most accurate food intake data; no memory error	Cost; time-consuming; high respondent burden; may cause alteration of usual eating patterns; participants require training & supervision; feasible only for small samples
Diet history	Find "usual" or "average" food & nutrient intakes over time by recall & food records	Provides more detailed information on usual intake which correlates better with long-term nutritional status measures	Time-consuming; requires interviewer training; difficulty of standardizing interviewer methodology; feasible for small sample only; reliability & validity problems; high respondent burden; high cost

Table 9. World Health Organization Recommended Daily Intakes for Moderately
Active Adults

Person	Calories	Protein (gms)	Thiamin (mg)	Riboflavin (mg)	Niacin (mg)	Vitamin A (mcg)	Vitamin C (mg)	Calcium (mg)	Iron (mg)
Woman	2,200	29*	0.9	1.3	14.5	750	30	400-500	14-28
Pregnant	2,550	38*	1.0	1.5	16.8	750	50	1,000-1,200	NA
Lactating	2,750	46*	1.1	1.7	18.2	1,200	50	1,000-1,200	NA
Man	3,000	37*	1.2	1.8	19.8	750	30	400-500	5-9

*as egg or milk protein

Source: Passmore et al. 1974

Table 10. Summary of Studies on Dietary Intake of Women in Developing Countries

Location	Sample	Year/Season	Measure	Calories	Protein (gms)	Thiamin (mg)	Riboflavin (mg)	Niacin (mg)	Vitamin A	Vitamin C (mg)	Calcium (mg)	Iron (mg)
AFRICA												
The Gambia[1]	Lactating women: N unknown	--	X̄	1600	--	--	0.4-0.6	--	100-750 mcg	--	--	--
The Gambia[2]	PW(33)	Mar-June	X̄	1620								
		July-Oct		1340								
		Nov-Dec		1420								
	LW(0-7 mos. same women)	Mar-June	X̄	1740								
		Jul-Oct		1370								
		Nov-Dec		1890								
Upper Volta[3]	Farmers: nonpregnant (14F)	Dec./Jan. end of harvest	X̄	1515*	animal 0.8* vegetable 44.8	--	--	--	--	--	--	--
	(11M)			2148*	animal 10.3* vegetable 57.5	--	--	--	--	--	--	--
ASIA												
Philippines[4]	Urban household survey: household heads (83M)	--	X̄ of individual adequacy ratio (intake/RDA)	81.7 83.4	81.4 97.3	50.3 52.3	64.9 74.6	89.2 99.6	31.3 36.2	60.8 63.5	62.3 81.7	77.8 171.0
	adult offspring (31F)(30M)			75.1 80.1	78.2 96.6	54.7 50.0	62.5 60.7	84.5 97.5	23.0 28.8	44.4 45.5	55.8 75.6	60.7 170.8
Philippines[5]	LW(21)		X̄	2175	66							
Philippines[6]	LW(74)		X̄	1599	49							
	PW(39)			1591	54							
India[7]	Low SES: pregnant (100) lactating (70) same women before pregnancy (100)	--	X̄ X̄ X̄	1815 1858 2152	44 42.7 49.8	-- -- --	-- -- --	-- -- --	-- -- --	-- -- --	374.4 299.1 390.5	18.2 22.5 20.9

continued

Table 10 continued

Location	Sample	Year/Season	Measure	Calories	Protein (gms)	Thiamin (mg)	Riboflavin (mg)	Niacin (mg)	Vitamin A	Vitamin C (mg)	Calcium (mg)	Iron (mg)
India[8]	Hospital clinic patients	March-July 1978										
	pregnant:											
	low SES (9)		X̄	1730	85	--	--	--	--	--	--	--
	mid SES (13)		X̄	1980	80	--	--	--	--	--	--	--
	high SES (9)		X̄	2100	86	--	--	--	--	--	--	--
	same women lactating:								β-carotene (mcg)			
	low SES (9)		X̄	2316	50	0.2	1.6	--	1593	2.5	1032	23
	mid SES (13)		X̄	2968	59	1.2	2.0	--	2444	8.4	1290	22
	high SES (9)		X̄	--	57	1.3	1.6	--	2185	5.6	1228	30
India[9]	LW;		X̄									
	very poor (54)			1439	39.6							
	poor (50)			1872	46.1							
	middle (57)			1906	47.2							
	upper middle (49)			2279	55.0							
India[10]	LW(24) low SES		X̄	1524	39.0							
India[11]	LW(20)		X̄	2961	65.0							
India[12]	LW(12); supplemental		X̄	1515	54.0							
India[13]	LW(39): 4 wks		X̄	1702	35.0							
	16 wks			2090	42.6							
	52 wks			1711	35.6							
New Guinea[14]	Subsistence farmers:	--			animal:							
	coastal:											
	pregnant (9)		X̄	1414	3.6	--	--	--	--	--	--	--
	lactating (13)		X̄	1412	3.0	--	--	--	--	--	--	--
	NPNL (34)		X̄	1402	3.1	--	--	--	--	--	--	--
	highlands:											
	pregnant (7)		X̄	2001	10.8	--	--	--	--	--	--	--
	lactating (14)		X̄	2133	9.2	--	--	--	--	--	--	--
	NPNL (14)		X̄	2068	10.4	--	--	--	--	--	--	--
Korea[15]	93 pregnant women; avg. SES, rural	winter 1976	X̄	2635	77.5	1.78	0.85	39.5	1235IU	87.2	491	14.7
			X̄ as % RDA	115%	82%	96%	51%	224%	52%	67%	41%	82%
			% < 66% RDA	4%	23%	1%	61%	0%	73%	16%	93%	31%
Micronesia[16]	43 women on wealthy, recently westernized Nauru Is.	Jan. 1976	X̄	5223	184	1.1	--	--	--	77	--	--

continued

Table 10 continued

Location	Sample	Year/Season	Measure	Calories	Protein (gms)	Thiamin (mg)	Riboflavin (mg)	Niacin (mg)	Vitamin A	Vitamin C (mg)	Calcium (mg)	Iron (mg)
Thailand[17]	Urban (15F)	--	X̄	1547	56	--	--	--	--	--	--	--
	(15M)		X̄	2013	63	--	--	--	--	--	--	--
	Rural (21M)		X̄	1292	46	--	--	--	--	--	--	--
	(21F)		X̄	1462	53	--	--	--	--	--	--	--
	(11 pregnant)		X̄	1980	39	1.57	0.89	17.2	1149IU	15.3	574	11.9
Singapore[18]	Random sample -- clinic patients: trimester 1 & 2 (14)	--	X̄	2386	57.1	1.1	0.8	14.3	1641mcg	--	365	11.0
	3 (23)		X̄	2487	69	1.3	1.0	15.4	1852mcg	113.5	419	12.4
	nonpregnant (24)		X̄	1927	53.2	0.9	0.9	11.5	1253mcg	70	--	9.5
LATIN AMERICA Guatemala[19]	Pregnant rural women, low SES:	--	X̄ as % RDA	64%	87%	90%	57%	--	36%	120%	171%	61%
				72%	83%	99%	55%	--	33%	58%	88%	61%
				76%	90%	107%	61%	--	47%	78%	92%	71%
Guatemala[20]	NPNL(=1st trimester)[20]		X̄	1418	39							
	PW, 3rd trimester(57)			1819	54							
	LW(36)			1599	58							
Guatemala[21]	LW(N unknown) supplemented: 3 mos.		X̄	1766	55.5							
	6 mos.			1764	55.2							
	9 mos.			1795	54.5							
	12 mos.			1708	54.0							
Guatemala[22]	NPNL(6) LW(18) both groups supplemented		X̄	1876	47.6							
				1929								
Guatemala[23]	Pregnant, 2d half (720) Lactating:	1969-77	X̄	1562±440	--	--	--	--	--	--	--	--
	3 mos. (520)			1766±573	--	--	--	--	--	--	--	--
	6 mos. (385)			1764±614	--	--	--	--	--	--	--	--
	9 mos. (381)			1795±590	--	--	--	--	--	--	--	--
	1 yr (372)			1708±558	--	--	--	--	--	--	--	--

Table 10 continued

Location	Sample	Year/season	Measure	Calories	Protein (gms)	Thiamin (mg)	Riboflavin (mg)	Niacin (mg)	Vitamin A	Vitamin C (mg)	Calcium (mg)	Iron (mg)
Brazil[24]	Random sample semiurban migrant workers: (94F)		X̄ as % FAO recommendation	1068 / 49%	28 / 68%	.41 / 46%	.40 / 31%	5.30 / 37%	172mcg / 23%	15 / 50%	170 / 43%	5.6 / 20%
	(76M)		X̄ as % FAO recommendation	2008 / 67%	51 / 96%	.76 / 63%	.68 / 38%	8.85 / 45%	248mcg / 33%	21.1 / 70%	251 / 63%	10.5 / 117%
Mexico[25]	Tarahumara Indians living traditional life in mountains (95F)	dry season 1973/74	X̄ as % FAO	2252	79	1.9 / 211%	1.1 / 85%	13.7 / 94%	1873mcg / 249%	84 / 280%	650 / 144%	25 / 89%
	(79M)		X̄ as % FAO	2818	92	2.2 / 183%	1.6 / 89%	17.8 / 90%	1881mcg / 251%	80 / 267%	726 / 161%	29 / 320%
Mexico[26]	Pregnant (42) lactating (12) NPNL (54)		X̄ / X̄ / X̄	2020 / 2030 / 1750	53.1 / 54.2 / 47.1	--	--	--	--	--	--	--
Puerto Rico[27]	Homemakers (109, including in at least 10 PW)		% > 100% RDA / 67-100% RDA / 34-66% RDA / ≤ 33% RDA	46 / 28 / 26 / 0	80 / 14 / 5 / 1		60 / 22 / 15 / 3		48 / 19 / 20 / 13	53 / 13 / 19 / 15	30 / 29 / 30 / 11	6 / 29 / 49 / 16
NEAR EAST												
Iraq[28]	Pregnant women, urban, low SES at MCH clinic < 5 mos (97), > 5 mos (60)	Fall 1963	X̄ as % RDA	79% / 85%	74% / 74%	76% / 73%	52% / 49%	52% / 56%	43% / 59%	33% / 39%	28% / 25%	52% / 59%
Egypt[29]	Rural trimester 1 (17) / 2 (19) / 3 (14)	--	% < 75% RDA	12% / 37% / 29%	0 / 37% / 7%	24% / 37% / 29%	53% / 74% / 57%	41% / 63% / 57%	--	18% / 26% / 21%	100% / 100% / 100%	70% / 75% / 93%

continued

Table 10 continued

Iran[30]

Outpatients at 2 urban hospitals; 3 mos after birth

low SES (15)	X̄	1840	61	1.4	1.0	--	29101U	32	506	15
	X̄ as % RDA	70%	90%	130%	60%	--	70%	105%	50%	55%
mid SES (28)	X̄	2270	82	1.7	1.5	--	71431U	80	788	18
	X̄ as % RDA	80%	120%	155%	85%	--	180%	265%	80%	65%

*significantly different

Notes: NPNL = nonpregnant, nonlactating
         FAO = Food and Agriculture Organization
         RDA = Recommended Dietary Allowances

Source: (1) Whitehead 1980; (2) Paul et al. 1979b; (3) Bleiberg et al. 1980; (4) Florencio & Aligaen 1980; (5) Villa-Real 1975;
          (6) N.; 1977 (7) Pasricha 1958; (8) Gupta & Sharma 1980; (9) Karmarkar et al. 1959;
          (10) Devadas & Mangalam 1970; (11) Devadas et al. 1978; (12) Devadas et al. 1971; (13) Sundararaj & Pereira 1975;
          (14) Durnin 1980; (15) KSA 1977; (16) Ringrose & Zimmet 1979; (17) Dhanamitta et al. c.1978; (18) Banerjee et al. 1972;
          (19) Demarchi et al. 1966; (20) Arroyave 1976; (21) Delgado et al. 1981; (22) Schultz et al. 1980; (23) Valverde et al.
          1981; (24) El-Sayed et al. 1980; (25) Geissler 1978; (26) Lechtig & Arroyave 1977; (27) Immink et al. 1981;
          (28) Desai et al. 1980; (29) Cerqueira et al. 1979; (30) Martinez et al. 1977

Table 11. Summary of Studies of Anthropometric Measurements of Women in Developing Countries

Study	Sample	Year/Season	Measure	Height (cm)	Weight (kg)	Triceps Skinfold (mm)	Arm Circum. (cm)	Arm Muscle Circum. (cm)	Weight for Height >90%	Weight for Height 81-90%	Weight for Height <80%
Reference Standards- Ten State Nutrition Survey, USA [1]	White women 25-35 yrs	--	5th %ile	--	--	9	23.0	17.7	--	--	--
			15th %ile	--	--	12	24.3	18.9	--	--	--
	white men 25-35 yrs		5th %ile	--	--	4	26.0	22.0	--	--	--
			15th %ile	--	--	6	28.0	24.1	--	--	--
AFRICA											
Upper Volta [2]	Farmers NP (14F) (11M)	Dec/Jan end of harvest	X̄ X̄	158 169	49.9 56.5	-- --	-- --	-- --	-- --	X̄=91% of standard X̄=80% of standard	
The Gambia [3]	NPNL (14) LW,4-36wks(62)	rainy season other season			wt. loss in both LW&NPNL LW maintained or gained wt.						
The Gambia [4]	LW,thru 3 mo(29)	rainy season other seasons			wt. loss gained wt., even at low intakes						
ASIA											
East Java [5]	Random sample large-scale nutrition survey NPNL (2150) lactating (1421)	1975-76 dry season	X̄ X̄	149 148	42.0 42.8	-- --	23.4 23.2	-- --	65% 77%	29% 21%	6% 2%
	pregnant: trimester 1 (59) 2 (83) 3 (104)		X̄ X̄ X̄	149 149 149	42.4 45.3 48.2	-- -- --	22.6 23.2 22.9	-- -- --	67% 59% 43%	25% 35% 46%	6% 6% 11%
Micronesia [6]	Residents of newly Westernized Nauru Is. (142F) (128M)		X̄ X̄	155.4 166.8	82.6 88.7	-- --	-- --	-- --	-- --	-- --	-- --

continued

Table 11 continued

Study	Sample	Year/ Season	Measure	Height (cm)	Weight (kg)	Triceps Skinfold (mm)	Arm Circum. (cm)	Arm Muscle Circum. (cm)	Weight for Height > 90%	81-90%	< 80%
Dominica[13]	PW(340)	1978	X̄, 1st visit (19.4 wks) last visit (37.8 wks)		60.2 kg 66.4 kg						
			X̄ % of reference wt., 1st visit last visit		95.3 94.0						
Guatemala[14]	LW(480-552) supplemented, at 12 mos		X̄, compared with: 1st trim. 3rd trim.		lost 0.90 kg lost 7.14 kg						
Guatemala[15]	Pregnant trimester 1 (265) 2 (274) 3 (400)		X̄ weight standardized by height		47.33±6.56 49.98±6.24 53.57±6.58	-- -- --	-- -- --	-- -- --	-- -- --	-- -- --	-- -- --
	lactating 3 mos (480) 6 mos (496) 9 mos (533) 1 yr (552)		X̄ weight standardized by height		48.39±6.16 47.67±6.23 47.05±6.27 46.43±5.87	-- -- -- --	-- -- -- --	-- -- -- --	-- -- -- --	-- -- -- --	-- -- -- --
Guatemala[16]	NPNL(6) LW(18), avg. 10 mos		X̄ X̄		← 35 gm/mo ← 369 gm/mo	-- --	-- --	-- --	-- --	-- --	-- --
Mexico[17]	Tarahumara Indians living traditional life in mountains women, age 19-30 (29) 31-50 (14) men, age 19-30 (41) 31-50 (37)		X̄	152 151 163 163	56 58 60 60	13 14 7 7	-- -- -- --	-- -- -- --	-- -- -- --	-- -- -- --	-- -- -- --

NEAR EAST

Table 11 continued

Study	Sample	Year/Season	Measure	Height (cm)	Weight (kg)	Triceps Skinfold (mm)	Arm Circum. (cm)	Arm Muscle Circum. (cm)	Weight for Height > 90%	81-90%	< 80%
New Guinea[7]	Subsistence farmers coastal:	--									
	pregnant (9)		x̄	153±6	51.7±7.0	--	--	--	--	--	--
	NP age 18-29 (29)		x̄	152±5	49.0±5.1	--	--	--	--	--	--
	NP age 30+ (31)		x̄	150±4	44.4±4.7	--	--	--	--	--	--
	highlands:										
	pregnant (7)		x̄	153±4	53.5±4.9	--	--	--	--	--	--
	NP age 18-29 (28)		x̄	152±5	51.3±6.1	--	--	--	--	--	--
	NP age 30+ (6)		x̄	150±4	45.8±5.2	--	--	--	--	--	--
New Guinea[8]	LW(153)				neg. assoc. with duration lactation						
India[9]	Urban pregnant trimester	--									
	1 (408)		x̄	150.8±4	44.3±5.4	--	22.6±2.42	--	--	--	--
	2 (1522)		x̄	150.1±5.3	47.1±5.8	--	21.3±2.1	--	--	--	--
	NPNL(1025)		x̄	150.1±5.2	44.4±8.2	--	23.0±2.6	--	--	--	--
	lactating										
	0-6 mos (860)		x̄	150.2±5.2	44.2±7.2	--	23.1±2.6	--	--	--	--
	7-12 mos (609)		x̄	149.4±7.1	42.9±6.7	--	22.3±2.6	--	--	--	--
India[10]	LW,supplemented (12)		x̄ wt.loss		1.79 kg						
	controls (12)				2.91 kg						
India[11]	LW,thru 6 mos(40) teenage adult		x̄ wt.loss		1.4 kg 0.3 kg						
LATIN AMERICA											
Brazil[12]	Random sample migrant families (85F)	--	x̄	153	57.0	14.3	27.6	23.1	80%	14.1%	5.9%
			x̄ as % standard	--	110%	87%	97%	100%	--	--	--
	(39M)	--	x̄	164	59.6	5.0	27.2	25.6	66.7%	23.1%	10.2%
			x̄ as % standard	--	95%	40%	93%	101%	--	--	--

continued

table 11 continued

Iran[18]											
Pregnant urban hospital outpatients	--										
low SES											
pregnant (36)	X̄	155	62.7	--	--	--	--	--	--	--	--
postpartum (21)	X̄	--	55.2	--	--	--	--	--	--	--	--
mid SES											
pregnant (52)	X̄	155	60.8	--	--	--	--	--	--	--	--
postpartum (36)	X̄	--	52.8	--	--	--	--	--	--	--	--
Jordan[19]											
NP women, ages	X̄										
20-24 (633)		154.7	58.7	--	--	--	--	--	--	--	--
25-29 (1022)		155.2	61.2	--	--	--	--	--	--	--	--
30-34 (736)		155.3	63.3	--	--	--	--	--	--	--	--
35-39 (527)		155.1	65.7	--	--	--	--	--	--	--	--
40-44 (264)		155.7	67.4	--	--	--	--	--	--	--	--

Notes: NP = nonpregnant; NPNL = nonpregnant, nonlactating

Source: (1) Frisancho 1974; (2) Bleiberg et al. 1980; (3) Thomson et al. 1966; (4) Paul et al. 1979b; (5) Kusin et al. 1979; (6) Ringrose & Zimmet 1979; (7) Durnin 1980; (8) Harrison et al. 1975; (9) NIN 1980; (10) Devadas et al. 1971; (11) Devadas et al. 1978; (12) Desai et al. 1980; (13) Gueri et al. 1982; (14) Delgado et al. 1981; (15) Valverde et al. 1981; (16) Schultz et al. 1980; (17) Cerqueira et al. 1979; (18) Geissler 1978; (19) Hijazi 1977

Table 12. Prevalence of Low Birth Weight in Several Developing Countries (percentage of births under 2,500 g)

Location	Area	Sample	1950-59	1960-69	1970-79
AFRICA[1]	All	20 million live births			15
Congo (Zaire)[1]	All			10-24.4	
Ethiopia[1]	All			16.5	8.8-16.5
Rhodesia[1]	All		16.6	11	
Sudan[1]	All			17.3	
			5-7		
			15.6		
			14		
Nigeria[1]		1,111 single normal pregnancies w/ pre-natal care, low SES			
		urban			9.4
		rural			9.8
ASIA[1]	All	72 million live births			20
Burma[3]	All				20
Singapore			21[1]	16.8[1]	11[3]
India[1]	New Delhi			40	
	Calcutta		34.7		
Korea[1]	All		10*		
Philippines[3]	All(estimate)				19.5
Philippines[2]				14.2	
Ceylon[4]		1,988 urban, hospital births			21
LATIN AMERICA[1]	All				11
Guatemala[1]	All			13.3	
Mexico[1]	Mexico City		11		
Puerto Rico[1]	All		8.9	9.8	9.2-9.4
NEAR EAST					
Syria[1]	All			19.9	
Israel[5]	Bedouins	1,959 hospital births			11.4
UNITED STATES	All				7.5
	Total White		6.9	7	6.4
	Total Nonwhite		11.6	12.5	12.5

*1959-60

Sources: (1) Boldman & Reed 1977; (2) Odutan & Ayeni 1974; (3) WHO 1980; (4) Soysa & Jayasuriya 1975; (5) Harlap et al. 1977.

Table 13. Summary of Maternal Supplementation Studies

Program	Description & Target	Impact on Maternal Nutrition Status	Unsupplemented Intake	Nutritional Content of Supplement	Type of Supplement	Distribution & Frequency	Period of Supplementation	Degree of Substitution
AFRICA								
Gambia[1]	Rural village; N unknown but probably 100 lactating women	↑723 kcal/day Wt. ↑ during lactation 1-2 kg	40-60% of caloric requirement 1100-1650 cal	950-1100 kcal/day	Locally prepared biscuit	On-site, 6 times/week	1 yr	↓Home intake by 107 cal/day
ASIA								
India Project Poshak, Exploratory Phase[2]	Integrated health & nutrition program; all pregnant & lactating women	Pregnant; ↑ 91 kcal/day Lactating: ↓ 200 kcal/day	Pregnant: 2400 kcal Lactating: 2600 kcal	754 cal 38 gm prot/ day	Instant corn soya milk	Take home, weekly	1 yr	NA
Taiwan[3]	294 low SES "marginally malnourished" rural mothers	Trimester 1: ↑ 389 cal 25 gm prot /day 2: ↑ 412 cal ↑ 38 gm prot /day 3: ↑ 484 cal ↑ 27 gm prot /day	1400 cal 40 gm prot	1. 800 kcal 40 gm prot/ day 2. 80 kcal/day	Canned liquid	Take home w/ strong outreach; twice daily	From birth of 1st infant through next pregnancy & next lactation	↓Home intake by 60-80 kcal/day
LATIN AMERICA								
Bogotá[4]	546 urban families w/ malnourished children & pregnant women; included health care	↑ 155 cal ↑ 20 gm prot/ day	1600 cal 36 gm prot	856 cal 38 gm prot/ family member	Powdered milk, bread, vegetables, oil	Last trimester of pregnancy	NA	
Guatamala[5]	651 low SES rural, pregnant women in 4 villages	↑ 235 kcal/day; significant increment correlation of supplementation with BW	1500 cal 40 gm prot	unrestricted	Gruel (atole) high cal/high prot; beverage (fresco) lower calorie	On site, twice daily	During pregnancy	Negative but insignificant correlation between supplement & home intake
Mexico[6]	39 pregnant women	↑ 450 kcal/day ↑ Wt. gain 4.5 kg ↑ BW-220 gms	1960 cal	260 cal/day	Powdered milk	NA	From day 45 of pregnancy through lactation	Apparent increase of home intake of 190 calories

continued

Table 13 continued

Program	Description & Target	Impact on Maternal Nutrition Status	Unsupplemented Intake	Nutritional Content of Supplement	Type of Supplement	Distribution & Frequency	Period of Supplementation	Degree of Substitution
Mexico-Food for Work[6]	Rural community food-for-work & nutrition education; N unknown; entire family	No long-term change in intake or introfamilial distribution	1700 kcal 54 gm prot	6000 kcal/ per family	Maize, beans, meat, fish, powdered milk (for pregnant & lactating women & children)	Take home, monthly	6 mos	NA
Peru[7]	Sample from 4 plantation villages w/ 3500 residents; N unknown; entire family	Changes in hts and wts of women independent of supplementation	NA	1. 250 kcal 7.5 gm prot 2. 250 kcal 12.5 gm prot	Noodles	Take home, weekly	5 yrs	Author feels high degree but no data

↑ increases

↓ decreases

Source: (1) Prentice et al 1980; (2) Gopaldas et al. 1975; (3) McDonald et al. c.1980; (4) Mora et al. 1979; (5) Lechtig et al. 1975; (6) Chavez et al. 1980; (7) Baertl et al. 1970.

Figure 1. Factors Affecting Women's Dietary Intake and Needs: A Conceptual Framework

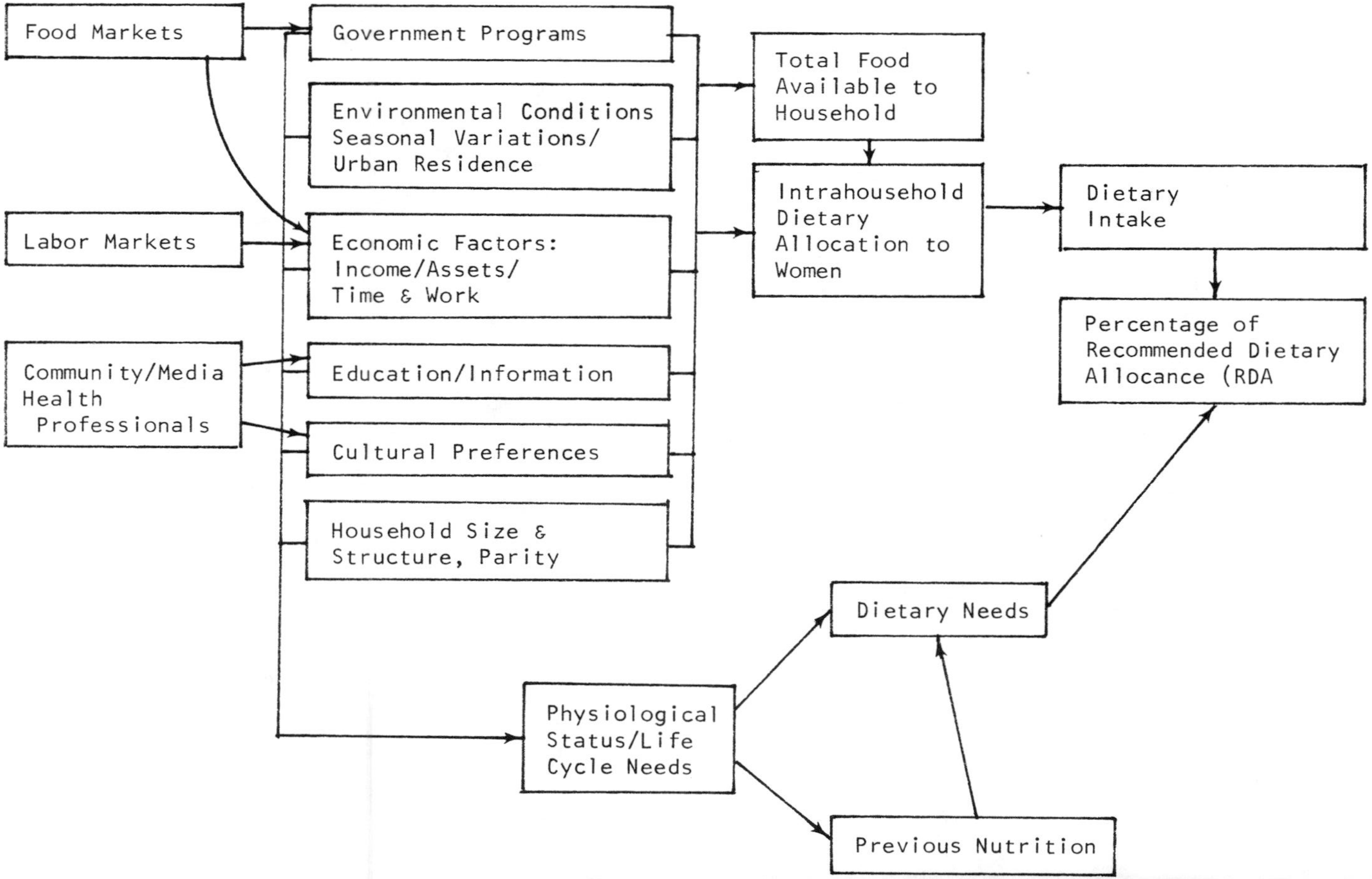

Selected Bibliography

Acharya, Meena. 1981. "Time Use Data from Nepalese Villages: Policy Implications." Paper presented at the Population Association of America, Washington, DC, March 28.

Adams, P. W.; Rose, David P.; Folkard, J.; Wynn, V.; Seed, M.; and Strong, R. 1973. "Effect of Pyridoxine Hydrochloride (Vitamin B6) upon Depression Associated with Oral Contraception." Lancet 1 (April 28): 897-904.

ADC. See Agricultural Development Council.

Agricultural Development Council. 1975. "Role of Women in Development." New York.

Ahmed, Faizy; Bamji, Mahtib S.; and Iyengar, Leela. 1975. "Effect of Oral Contraceptive Agents on Vitamin Nutrition Status." American Journal of Clinical Nutrition 28: 606-15.

Akin, John S.; Guilkey, David K.; and Popkin, Barry M. 1981. "The Demand for Child Health Services in the Philippines." Social Science and Medicine 15C: 249-57.

Alvarez, Hermogenes; Vera-Medrano, Cesar; Sala, Miguel A.; and Benedetti, Washington L. 1972. "Trophoblast Development Gradient and Its Relationship to Placental Hemodynamics." American Journal of Obstetrics and Gynecology 114: 873-78.

American Public Health Association. 1977. The State of the Art of Delivering Low Cost Health Services in Developing Countries. Washington, DC.

Annegers, John F. 1973. "Seasonal Food Shortages in West Africa." Ecology of Food and Nutrition 2: 251-57.

Antonov, A. N. 1947. "Children Born during the Siege of Leningrad in 1942." Journal of Pediatrics 30: 250-59.

Aono, Toshihiro; Shioji, Takenori; Shoda, Tsuneo; and Kurachi, Keiichi. 1977. "The Initiation of Human Lactation and Prolactin Response to Sucking." Journal of Clinical Endocrinology and Metabolism 44: 1101-06.

APHA. See American Public Health Association.

Arroyave, Guillermo. 1976. "Nutrition in Pregnancy. Studies in Central America and Panama." Separata de Archives Latinoamericanos de Nutricion 26: 129-57.

Arroyave, Guillermo; Beghin, Ivan; Flores, Marina; DeGuido, Cecelia Soto; and Ticas, Jose María. 1974. "Efectos del consumo de azúcar fortificada con retinol por la madre embarazada y lactante cuja dieta habitual es en vitamina A. Estudio de la madre y del niño." Archivos

Latinoamericanos de Nutricion 24: 485-512.

Austin, James E. 1978. "The Perilous Journey of Nutrition Evaluation." American Journal of Clinical Nutrition 31:2324-38.

_____ 1980. Confronting Urban Malnutrition: The Design of Nutrition Programs. A World Bank Staff Occasional Paper, no. 28. Baltimore: Johns Hopkins University Press.

_____ 1981. "The Integration of Nutrition and Population Programs." In Nutrition Programs in the Third World: Cases and Concepts, edited by James E. Austin. Cambridge, MA: Oelgeschlager, Gunn & Hain, pp. 319-28.

Austin, James E.; Anderson, Mary Ann; Goldman, Richard; Heimendinger, Jerianne; Overholt, Catherine; Pyle, David; Rogers, Beatrice; Wray, Joe D.; and Zeitlin, Marian F. 1978a. Nutrition Intervention Assessment and Guidelines. Report to United Nations ACC Sub-Committee on Nutrition. Cambridge, MA: Harvard Institute for International Development.

Austin, James E.; Belding, Thomas K.; Brooks, Richard; Cash, Richard; Fisher, Jonathan; Morrow, Richard; Pielemeyer, Nancy; Pyle, David; Wray, Joe D.; and Zeitlin, Marian F. 1981a Nutrition Intervention in Developing Countries. Vol. 5. Study VII: Integrated Nutrition and Primary Health Care Programs. Cambridge, MA: Oelgeschlager, Gunn & Hain.

Austin, James E.; Belding, Thomas K.; Pyle, David; Solon, Florentino S.; Fernandez, Thomas L.; Latham, Michael C.; and Popkin, Barry M. 1981b. Nutrition Intervention in Developing Countries. Vol. 3. Study III: Fortification. Cambridge, MA: Oelgeschlager, Gunn & Hain.

Austin, James E.; Mahin, Melanie; Pyle, David; and Zeitlin, Marian F. 1978a. Annotated Directory of Nutrition Programs in Developing Countries. Cambridge, MA: Harvard Institute for International Development.

Ayres, Barbara. 1967. "Pregnancy Magic: A Study of Food Taboos and Sex Avoidances." In Cross-Cultural Approaches. Readings in Comparative Research, edited by Clellan Stearns Ford. New Haven: Human Relations Area File Press, pp. 111-25.

Baertl, Juan M.; Morales, Enrique; Verastegui, Gustavo; and Graham, George G. 1970. "Diet Supplementation for Entire Communities: Growth and Mortality of Infants and Children." American Journal of Clinical Nutrition 23: 707-15.

Baldwin, Robert E. and Weisbrod, Burton A. 1974. "Diseases and Labor Productivity." Economic Development and Cultural Change 22: 414-35.

Banerjee, B.; Khew, K.S.; and Saha, N. 1971. "A Comparative Study of Energy Expenditure in Some Common Daily Activities of Non-pregnant and Pregnant Chinese, Malay and Indian Women." The Journal of Obstetrics and Gynecology of the British Commonwealth 78: 113-16.

Banerjee, B.; Tan, P.Y.; and Saha, N. 1972. "Calorie and Nutrient Intake of Pregnant Asian Women." Tropical and Geographical Medicine 24: 249-52.

Barsivala, Villi M. and Virkar, Katayun D. 1973. "The Effect of Oral Contraceptives on Concentrations of Various Components of Human Milk." Contraception 7: 307-12.

Basson, Priscilla, 1982. "Domestic Productivity in Male-and Female-Headed Households in Rural Jordan." Ecology of Food and Nutrition 12: 75-78.

Basta, Samir S. 1977. "Nutrition and Health in Low Income Urban Areas of the Third World." Ecology of Food and Nutrition 6: 113-24.

Basta, Samir S. and Churchill, Anthony. 1974. "Iron Deficiency Anemia and the Productivity of Adult Males in Indonesia." World Bank Staff Working Paper, no. 175. Washington, DC: International Bank for Reconstruction and Development.

Battad, Josephine. 1979. "Determinants of Nutritional Status in Rural Philippine Households." In Rural Asian Household Studies, edited by Hans P. Binswanger, Robert E. Evenson, Cecelia A. Florencio, and Benjamin N.F. White. Singapore: Singapore University Press.

Bauer, Janet. 1979. "Demographic Change, Information Control, and Inter-generational Conflict in Iran." Paper presented to the 17th International Seminar on the Child and the Family, sponsored by the Committee on Family Research, International Sociological Association, Helsinki, Finland, November 26-30.

_____ 1981. "Changes in the Behavior and Consciousness of Iranian Women (1963-1978): A Structural Application of Social Learning Theory." Ph.D. dissertation, Stanford University.

Beaton, George H. and Bengoa, J.M. 1976. "Practical Population Indicators of Health and Nutrition." In Nutrition in Preventive Medicine: The Major Deficiency Syndromes, Epidemiology, and Approaches to Control, edited by George H. Beaton and J. M. Bengoa. World Health Organization Monograph Series, no. 62. Geneva, pp. 500-19.

Beaton, George H. and Ghassemi, H. 1983. "Supplementary Feeding Programs for Young Children in Developing Countries." American Journal of Clinical Nutrition 37 (supp.): 864-916.

Beck, Lois Grant. 1978. "Women Among Qashga'i Nomadic Pastoralists in Iran." In Women in the Muslim World, edited by Lois Grant Beck and Nikki Keddie. Cambridge, MA: Harvard University Press, pp. 351-73.

Becker, Stan and Sardar, M.A. 1978. "Seasonal Patterns of Vital Events in Matlab Thana, Bangladesh." In Seasonal Dimensions to Rural Poverty, edited by Robert Chambers, Richard Longhurst, and Arnold Pacey. London: Pinter; Totowa, NJ: Allanheld, Osmun, pp. 149-54.

Beenstock, Michael. 1978. "Nutrition and Productivity." [Washington, DC: International Bank for Reconstruction and Development.]

Beisel, W.R.; Edelman, R.; Nauss, K.; and Suskind, R.M. 1981. "Single-Nutrient Affects on Immunologic Functions." Journal of the American Medical Association 245: 53-58.

Belavady, B. 1966. "Nutrition and Efficiency in Agricultural Labourers." Indian Journal of Medical Research 54: 971-76.

Bell, R.M.S.; Daly, J.; Kanengoni, E.; and Jones, J.J. 1973. "The Effects of Endemic Schistosomiasis and of Hycanthone on the Mental Ability of African School Children." Transactions of the Royal Society of Tropical Medicine and Hygiene 67: 694-701.

Belsey, Mark A. 1977. "Hormonal Contraception and Nutrition." In Nutrition Impacts on Women Throughout Life with Emphasis on Reproduction, edited by Kamran S. Moghissi and Tommy N. Evans. Hagerstown, MD: Harper & Row, pp. 189-200.

Berg, Alan with Muscat, R.J. 1973. The Nutrition Factor: Its Role in National Development. Washington, DC: The Brookings Institution.

Bergner, Lantence and Susser, Mervyn W. 1970. "Low Birth Weight and Prenatal Nutrition, An Interpretative Review." Pediatrics 46: 946-66.

Bierman, Edwin L. 1979. "Carbohydrate, Sucrose, and Human Disease." American Journal of Clinical Nutrition 32: 2712-22.

Billewicz, W.Z.; Fellowes, H.M.; and Hytten, C.A. 1976. "Comments on the Critical Metabolic Mass and the Age of Menarche." Annals of Human Biology 3: 51-59.

Birdsall, Nancy. 1980. "Measuring Time Use and Nonmarket Exchange." In Third World Poverty: New Strategies for Measuring Development Progress, edited by William Paul McGreevey. The Battelle Human Affairs Research Centers Series. Cambridge, MA: Lexington Books, pp. 157-74.

Birdsall, Nancy and McGreevey, William Paul. 1983. "Women, Poverty and Development. In Women and Poverty in the Third World, edited by Mayra Buvinic, Margaret A. Lycette, and William Paul McGreevey. Baltimore: Johns Hopkins University Press, pp. 3-13.

Blackwell, R. Quentin; Chow, Bacon F.; Chinn, Kenneth S.K.; Blackwell, Boon-Nam; and Hsu, S.C. 1973. "Prospective Maternal Nutrition Study in Taiwan: Rationale, Study Design, Feasibility, and Preliminary Findings."

Nutrition Reports International 7: 517-32.

Blair, Patricia. 1980. "Programming for Women and Health." Paper prepared for the Office of Women in Development, Bureau of Programs and Policy Coordination, Agency for International Development, Washington, DC.

Bleiberg, Fanny M.; Brun, Thierry A.; Goihman, Samuel; and Gouba, Emile. 1980. "Duration of Activities and Energy Expenditure of Female Farmers in Dry and Rainy Seasons in Upper Volta." British Journal of Nutrition 43: 71-82.

Blumberg, Rae Lesser. 1976. "Fairy Tales and Facts: Economy, Family, Fertility, and the Female." In Women and World Development, With an Annotated Bibliography, edited by Irene Tinker, Michèle Bo Bramsen, and Mayra Buvinić. Praeger Special Studies in International Economics and Development. New York: Praeger, pp. 12-21.

Boldman, Rosanne and Reed, Dwayne M. 1977. "Worldwide Variations in Low Birth Weight." In The Epidemiology of Prematurity, edited by Dwayne M. Reed and Fiona J. Stanley. Baltimore: Urban & Schwarzenberg, pp. 39-51.

Bolton, J. M. 1972. "Food Taboos Among the Orang Asli in West Malaysia: A Potential Nutritional Hazard." American Journal of Clinical Nutrition 25: 789-99.

Bongaarts, John. 1980. "Does Malnutrition Affect Fecundity? A Summary of Evidence." Science 208 (May 9): 564-69.

Bongaarts, John and Delgado, Hernán. 1979. "Effects of Nutritional Status on Fertility in Rural Guatemala." In Natural Fertility: Patterns and Determinants of Natural Fertility. Proceedings of a Seminar on Natural Fertility, edited by Henri Leridon and Jane A. Menken. Liege: Ordina Editions, pp. 107-33.

Borazjani, Gholamreza; Javey, Houshang; Sadjadi, Hasan E.; and Daneshbod, Khosrow. 1978. "Maternal Mortality in South Iran: A Seven-Year Survey." International Journal of Gynaecology and Obstetrics 16: 65-69.

Borglin, Nils-Erik and Sandholm, Lars-Erik. 1971. "Effect of Oral Contraceptives on Lactation." Fertility and Sterility 22: 39-41.

Bornstein, Annika and Kreysler, Joachim. 1972. "Social Factors Influencing Attendance in 'Under-Fives' Clinics." Journal of Tropical Pediatrics and Environmental Child Health 18: 150-57.

Boserup, Ester. 1970. Women's Role in Economic Development. London: Allen & Unwin.

Bradbury, A. J. 1977. "Congenital Malaria in One Non-identical Twin." British Medical Journal 2 (September 3): 613.

Bradley, David. 1981. "Seasonal Variables in Infective Disease: A Summary." In Seasonal Dimensions to Rural Poverty, edited by Robert Chambers, Richard Longhurst, and Arnold Pacey. London: Pinter; Totowa, NJ: Allanheld, Osmun, pp. 127-33.

Brasel, Jo Anne. 1978. "Impact of Malnutrition on Reproductive Endocrinology." In Nutrition and Human Reproduction, edited by W. Henry Mosley. New York: Plenum, pp. 29-60.

Bray, R. S. 1981. "Insect-Borne Diseases: Malaria." In Seasonal Dimensions to Rural Poverty, edited by Robert Chambers, Richard Longhurst, and Arnold Pacey. London: Pinter; Totowa, NJ: Allanheld, Osmun, pp. 116-20.

Briend, Andre. 1980. "Maternal Physical Activity, Birthweight, and Perinatal Mortality." Medical Hypothesis 6: 1157-70.

Briggs, Maxine. 1976. "Biochemical Effects of Oral Contraceptives." Advances in Steroid Biochemistry and Pharmacology 5: 65-160.

Brimblecombe, F.S.W.; Ashford, J.R.; and Fryer, J.G. 1968. "Significance of Low Birth Weight in Perinatal Mortality: A Study of Variations Within England and Wales." British Journal of Preventive and Social Medicine 22: 27-35.

Briscoe, John. 1978. "The Role of Water Supply in Improving Health in Poor Countries (with Special Reference to Bangladesh)." American Journal of Clinical Nutrition 31: 2100-13.

Brun, Thierry A.; Bleiberg, Fanny M.; and Goihman, Samuel. 1981. "Energy Expenditure of Male Farmers in Dry and Rainy Seasons in Upper-Volta." British Journal of Nutrition 45: 67-75.

Bruton, Henry J. 1980. "Employment Growth as an Indication of Poverty Alleviations." In Third World Poverty, edited by William Paul McGreevey. Human Affairs Research Center Series. Cambridge, MA: Lexington Books.

Buchanan, Robert. 1975. "Effects of Childbearing on Maternal Health." Population Reports, Ser. J, no. 8: 125-40.

Burelle, R.J.W.; Healey, M.J.R.; and Tanner, J.M. 1961. "Age at Menarche in South African Bantu Schoolgirls Living in Transkei Reserve." Human Biology 33: 250-61.

Buvinič, Mayra with Adams, Cheri S.; Edgcomb, Gabrielle S.; and Koch-Weser, Maritta. 1976. Women and World Development: An Annotated Bibliography. Washington, DC: Overseas Development Council.

Buvinič, Myra and Youssef, Nadia Haggag with Von Elm, Barbara. 1978. Women-Headed Households: The Ignored Factor in Development Planning. Reports Submitted to AID/WID. Washington, DC: International Center for Research on Women.

Cain, Mead; Khanam, Syeda Rokeya; and Nahar, Shamsun. 1979. "Class, Patriarchy, and Women's World in Bangladesh." Population and Development Review 5: 405-38.

Cassel, John. 1971. "Health Consequences of Population Density and Crowding." In Rapid Population Growth: Consequences and Policy Indicators, prepared by a Study Committee of the Office of the Foreign Secretary, National Academy of Sciences with the Support of the Agency for International Development. Baltimore: Johns Hopkins University Press for the National Academy of Sciences, pp. 462-78.

Castelazao-Ayalia, L. 1971. "Aetiological Factors of Anemia During Pregnancy: Observations in Latin American Countries." In Proceedings of the International Seminar on Maternal Mortality, Family Planning and Biology of Reproduction, edited by B. N. Purandare and C. L. Jhaveri. Bombay, pp. 58-64.

Cerqueira, Maria T.; Fry, Martha McMurry; and Connor, William E. 1979. "The Food and Nutrient Intakes of the Tarahumara Indians of Mexico." American Journal of Clinical Nutrition 32: 905-15.

Chambers, Robert. 1979. "Health, Agriculture, and Rural Poverty: Why Seasons Matter." Discussion Paper, no. 148. Brighton, England: Institute of Development Studies, University of Sussex.

Chambers, Robert; Longhurst, Richard; Bradley, David; and Feachem, Richard. 1979. "Seasonal Dimensions to Rural Poverty: Analysis and Practical Implications." Discussion Paper, no. 142. Brighton England: Institute of Development Studies, University of Sussex.

Chase, Helen C. 1969. "Infant Mortality and Weight at Birth: 1960 United States Birth Cohort." American Journal of Public Health 59: 1618-28.

Chávez, Adolfo. 1978. "Effects of Malnutrition on Infant Body Morphology." In Birthweight Distribution: An Indication of Social Development, edited by G. Sterby and L. Mollander. Uppsala, Sweden, pp. 18-20.

Chávez, Adolfo and Martínez, Celia. 1975. "Nutrition and Development of Children from Poor Rural Areas. V. Nutrition and Behavioral Development." Nutrition Reports International 11: 477-89.

Chávez, Adolfo; Martínez, Celia; and Bourges, Hector. 1976. "Role of Lactation in the Nutrition of Low Socio-economic Groups." Ecology of Food and Nutrition 4: 159-69.

Chávez, Adolfo; Martínez, Celia; and Schlaepter, Loraine. 1980. "Health Effects of Supplemental Feeding Programs." Paper presented to the Western Hemisphere Congress of Nutrition, Los Angeles, August 11-14.

Chen, Lincoln C.; Ahmed, Shamsa; Gesche, Melita; and Mosley, W. Henry. 1974. "A Prospective Study of Birth Interval Dynamics in Rural Bangladesh." Population Studies 28: 277-97.

Chen, Lincoln C.; Chowdhury, A. K. M. Alauddin; and Huffman, Sandra L. 1979. "Seasonal Dimensions of Energy Protein Malnutrition in Rural Bangladesh; The Role of Agriculture, Dietary Practices, and Infection." Ecology of Food and Nutrition 8: 174-87.

Chen, Lincoln C.; Huq, Emdadul; and D'Souza, Stan. 1981. "Sex Bias in the Family Allocation of Food and Health Care in Rural Bangladesh." Population and Development Review 7: 55-70.

Chernichovsky, Dov and Kielmann, Arnfried. 1978. "Socioeconomic Status, Diet, and Growth of Preschool Children in Rural Punjab--India." [Washington, DC: International Bank for Reconstruction and Development.]

Chowdhury, A. K. M. Alauddin. 1978. "Effect of Maternal Nutrition on Fertility in Rural Bangladesh." In Nutrition and Human Reproduction, edited by W. Henry Mosley. New York: Plenum, pp. 401-11.

Chowdhury, A. K. M. Alauddin; Huffman, Sandra L.; and Chen, Lincoln C. 1981. "Interaction of Agriculture, Dietary Practices, and Infection on Seasonal Dimensions of Energy Malnutrition." Paper presented to the Seasonal Dimensions to Rural Poverty Conference, University of Sussex, Brighton, England, July 3-6.

Chowdhury, A. K. M. Alauddin; Huffman, Sandra L.; and Curlin, George T. 1977. "Malnutrition, Menarche, and Marriage in Rural Bangladesh." Social Biology 24: 316-25.

Christiansen, Niels; Mora, J. O.; de Navarro, L.; and Herrera, M. G. 1980. "Effects of Nutritional Supplementation During Pregnancy Upon Birth Weight: The Influence of Pre-Supplementation Diet." Nutrition Reports International 21: 615-24.

Colle, Royal D. and Fernández de Colle, Susana. 1978. "The Communication Factor in Health and Nutrition Programmes: A Case Study from Guatemala." Cajanus 11: 151-96.

Council for Social Development. 1976. The Mahbubnager Experiment: Non-Formal Education for Rural Women. New Delhi: United Nations International Children's Emergency Fund.

Cravioto, Joaquin and DeLicardie, Elsa R. 1973. "The Effect of Malnutrition on the Individual." In Nutrition, National Development, and Planning: Proceedings of an International Conference Held at Cambridge, Massachusetts, October 19-21, 1971, edited by Alan Berg, Nevin S. Scrimshaw, and David L. Call. Cambridge, MA: MIT Press, pp. 3-21.

Crisp, A. H. and Stonehill, Edward. 1971. "Relation Between Aspects of Nutritional Disturbance and Menstrual Activity in Primary Anorexia Nervosa." British Medical Journal 3 (July 7): 149-51.

CSD. See Council for Social Development.

Dahl, Lewis K. 1972. "Salt and Hypertension." American Journal of Clinical Nutrition 25: 231-44.

DaVanzo, Julie and Lee, Donald Lye Poh. 1983. "The Compatability of Child Care with Nonmarket Activities: Preliminary Evidence from Malaysia." In Women and Poverty in the Third World, edited by Mayra Buvinić, Margaret A. Lycette, and William Paul McGreevey. Baltimore: Johns Hopkins University Press, pp. 62-91.

Davies, A. Michael. 1971. "Geographical Epidemiology of the Toxemias of Pregnancy." Israel Journal of Medical Sciences 7: 751-821.

Delgado, Hernán; Brineman, Elena; Lechtig, Aaron; Bongaarts, John; Martorell, Reynaldo; and Klein, Robert E. 1979. "Effect of Maternal Nutritional Status and Infant Supplementation During Lactation on Postpartum Amenorrhea." American Journal of Obstetrics and Gynecology 135: 303-07.

Delgado, Hernán; Lechtig, Aaron; Brineman, Elena; Martorell, Reynaldo;

Yarbrough, Charles; and Klein, Robert E. 1978. "Nutrition and Birth Interval Components: The Guatemalan Experience." In Nutrition and Human Reproduction, edited by W. Henry Mosley. New York: Plenum, pp. 385-99.

Delgado, Hernán; Lechtig, Aaron; Yarbrough, Charles; Martorell, Reynaldo; Klein, Robert E.; and Irwin, Marc. 1977. "Maternal Nutrition--Its Effects on Infant Growth and Development and Birthspacing." In Nutritional Impacts on Women Throughout Life with Emphasis on Reproduction, edited by Kamran S. Moghissi and Tommy N. Evans. Hagerstown, MD: Harper & Row, pp. 133-50.

Delgado, Hernán L.; Valverde, Victor E.; Martorell, Reynaldo; and Klein, Robert E. 1982. "Relationship of Maternal and Infant Nutrition to Infant Growth." Early Human Development 6: 273-86.

Delvoye, Pierre; Badawi, Mohamed; Demaegd, Marc; and Robyn, Claude. 1978. "Long-Lasting Lactation Is Associated with Hyperprolactinemia and Amenorrhea." In Progress in Prolactin Physiology and Pathology: Proceedings of the International Symposium on Prolactin, Nice, France, October 1977, edited by Claude Robyn and M. Harter. Developments in Endocrinology, vol. 2. Amsterdam: Elsevier/North Holland Biomedical Press, pp. 213-32.

Delvoye, Pierre; Delogne-Desnoeck, J.; and Robyn, Claude. 1976. "Serum-Prolactin in Long-Lasting Lactation Amenorrhea." The Lancet 2 (7 August): 288-89.

Delvoye, Pierre; Delgone-Desnoeck, J.; and Robyn, Claude. 1977. "The Influence of the Frequency of Nursing and of Previous Lactation Experience on Serum Prolactin in Lactating Mothers." Journal of Biosocial Science 9: 447-51.

Demarchi, M.; Isa, A.; Al-Saidi, S.; Al-Azzawee, M.; Ali, M.; and Elmilli, N. 1966. "Food Consumption and Nutrition Status of Pregnant Women Attending a Maternal Child Health Centre in Baghdad." Journal of the Faculty of Medicine-Baghdad 8: 20-30.

Deodhar, A. D. and Ramakrishnan, C. V. 1960. "Studies on Human Lactation. (Relationship Between the Dietary Intake of Lactating Women and the Chemical Composition of Milk with Regard to Vitamin Content)." Journal of Tropical Pediatrics and African Child Health 6: 44-47.

Deodhar, A. D.; Rajalakshmi, R.; and Ramakrishnan, C. V. 1964. "Studies on Human Lactation. Part 3. Effect of Dietary Supplementation on Vitamin Content of Breast Milk." Acta Paediatrica 53: 42-48.

Desai, I. D.; Garcia Tavares, M. L.; Dutra de Oliveria, B. S.; Douglas, A.; Duarte, F. A. M.; and Dutra de Oliveria, J. E. 1980. "Food Habits and Nutritional Status of Agricultural Migrant Workers in Southern Brazil." American Journal of Clinical Nutrition 33: 702-14.

Devadas, Rajammal P. and Mangalam, N. 1970. "The Nutritional Status of Nursing Mothers in a Village." Indian Journal of Nutrition and Dietetics 7: 153-59.

Devadas, Rajammal P.; Anuradha, J. R. Baby; and Sharadambal, B. 1971. "Evaluation of an Applied Nutrition Feeding Programme on the Nutritional Status of Nursing Women." Indian Journal of Nutrition and Dietetics 8: 143-48.

Devadas, Rajammal P.; Vijayalakshmi, P.; and Nagalakschmi, P. 1978. "Nutritional Profile of Selected Nursing Mothers in Coimbatore City." Indian Journal of Nutrition and Dietetics 15: 367-70.

Dhanamita, Sakorn; Sauvanus, Prasert; Tankeyura, Channeun; and Nimmannitaya, Suchon. c. 1978. Thailand--Country Reports on Food Habits, National Nutrition Problems, National Plan on Food and Nutrition Development. [Bangkok: Institute of Nutrition, Mahidol University.]

Dixon, Ruth B. 1980. Assessing the Impact of Development Projects on Women. AID Program Evaluation Discussion Paper, no. 8. Washington, DC: Office of Women in Development and Office of Evaluation, Bureau for Program and Policy Coordination, U.S. Agency for International Development.

Drake, William D.; Miller, Roy L.; and Humphrey, Margaret. 1980. Project on Analysis of Community-Level Nutrition Programs. Vol. 1. Final Report: Analysis of Community-Level Nutrition Programs. Washington, DC: U.S. Agency for International Development; Ann Arbor: Community Systems Foundation.

Drillien, C.M. 1974. "Prenatal and Perinatal Factors in Etiology and Outcome of Low Birth Weight." Clinics in Perinatology 1 (2): 197-211.

Ducommun, Rosalie. 1980. "The Old Barriers Remain." In "World Conference of the United Nations Decade for Women: Equality, Development and Peace." Development Forum (June, suppl.): (3).

Durnin, John Valentine George Andrew. 1976. "Sex Differences in Energy Intake and Expenditure." Proceedings of the Nutrition Society 35: 145-54.

_____. 1980. "Food Consumption and Energy Balance During Pregnancy and Lactation in New Guinea." In Maternal Nutrition During Pregnancy and Lactation: A Nestlé Foundation Workshop, Lutry/Lausanne, April 26th and 27th 1979, edited by Harry Aebi and Roger G. Whitehead. Nestlé Foundation Publication Series, no. 1. Bern: Hans Huber, pp. 86-95.

Durnin, John Valentine George Andrew and Passmore, Reginald. 1967. Energy, Work and Leisure. London: Heinemann.

Dyson, Tim and Crook, Nigel. 1981. "Causes of Seasonal Fluctuation in Vital Events." In Seasonal Dimensions of Rural Poverty, edited by Robert Chambers, Richard Longhurst, and Arnold Pacey. London: Pinter; Totowa, NJ: Allanheld, Osmun, pp. 135-41.

Eastman, Nicholas J. and Jackson, Esther. 1968. "Weight Relationships in Pregnancy. I. The Bearing of Maternal Weight Gain and Pre-Pregnancy Weight on Birth Weight in Full Term Pregnancies." Obstetrical and Gynecological Survey 23: 1003-25.

Edgerton, V. Reggie; Gardner, Gerald W.; Ohira, Y.; Gunawardena, K. A.; and Senewiratne, Brian. 1979. "Iron-Deficiency Anemia and Its Effect on Worker Productivity and Activity Patterns." British Medical Journal 2 (December 15): 1546-49.

Edozien, Joseph C.; Switzer, Boyd R.; and Bryan, Rebecca B. 1979. "Medical Evaluation of the Supplemental Food Program for Women, Infants, and Children." American Journal of Clinical Nutrition 32: 677-92.

el-Messiri, Sawsan. 1978. "Self-Images of Traditional Urban Women in Cairo." In Women in the Muslim World, edited by Lois Beck and Nikki Keddie. Cambridge, MA: Harvard University Press, pp. 522-40.

El-Sayed, Hekmat; Anine, Ezzat K.; and Shaheen, F. 1980. "Epidemiological Study of Anemias in Pregnancy in a Rural Community. Part I. Hematological, Biochemical and Dietary Studies." Cairo: Nutrition Institute.

Engle, Patricia L. 1980. "The Intersecting Needs of Working Women and Their Young Children: A Report to the Ford Foundation." [San Luis Obispo, CA: California Polytechnic State University.]

Evenson, Robert E. [1979] "The Allocation of Time by Adult Women: An International Comparison." [New Haven: Department of Economics, Yale University.]

Evenson, Robert E. and King-Quizon, Elizabeth. 1978. "Time Allocation and Home Production in Philippine Rural Households." Paper presented to the International Center for Research on Women Workshop on "Women in Poverty: What Do We Know?", Elkridge, MD, April 30-May 2.

Evenson, Robert E.; Popkin, Barry M.; and King-Quizon, Elizabeth. 1979. "Nutrition, Work and Demographic Behavior in Rural Philippine Households: A Synopsis of Several Laguna Household Studies." In Rural Asian Household Studies, edited by Hans P. Binswanger, Robert E. Evenson,

Cecelia A. Florencio, and Benjamin N. F. White. Singapore: Singapore University Press.

FAO. See Food and Agriculture Organization.

Farid, Z.; Bassily, S.; Schulert, A. R.; Zeind, A. S.; McConnell, E.; and Abdel Wahab, M. F. 1968. "Urinary Blood Loss in Schistosoma Haematobium Infection in Egyptian Farmers." Transactions of the Royal Society of Tropical Medicine and Hygiene 62: 496-500.

Farouk, A. and Ali, Muhammad. 1975. The Hardworking Poor: A Survey of How People Use Their Time in Bangladesh. Dacca, Bangladesh: Bureau of Economic Research, Dacca University.

Fedrick, Jean and Adlestein, Philippa A. 1978. "Factors Associated with Low Birth Weight of Infants Delivered at Term." British Journal of Obstetrics and Gynecology 85: 1-7.

Fernandez, W. 1971. "Analysis of Maternal Deaths Due to Anaemia in a General Hospital." In Proceedings of the International Seminar on Maternal Mortality, Family Planning and Biology of Reproduction, edited by B. N. Purandare and C. L. Jhaveri. Bombay, pp. 287-92.

Fiedler, John; Caldwell, Holly; Campbell, Claudia; and Dunlop, David W. 1978. "The Dynamics of Human Capital Formation in Developing Countries: A Review of the Relationship between Health, Nutrition, Education, and Population Change." Paper presented to the African Studies Association, Baltimore, November.

Filer, Lloyd J., Jr. 1977. "Relationship of Nutrition to Lactation and Newborn Development." In Nutritional Impacts on Women Throughout Life with Emphasis on Reproduction, edited by Kamran S. Moghissi and Tommy N. Evans. Hagerstown, MD: Harper & Row, pp. 151-59.

Florencio, Cecilia A. and Aligaen, Melba B. 1980. "Food and Nutrient Distribution in Filipino Urban Households." Nutrition Reports International 21: 375-85.

Florencio, Cecilia A. and Smith, Victor E. 1969. "Efficiency of Food Purchasing Among Working-Class Families in Colombia." Journal of the American Dietetic Association 55: 239-45.

Florey, Charles Du V.; McDonald, H.; McDonald, J.; and Miall, W. E. 1972. "The Prevalence of Diabetes in a Rural Population of Jamaican Adults." International Journal of Epidemiology 1: 157-66.

Food and Agriculture Organization. 1971. Energy and Protein Requirements. Report of a Joint FAO/WHO Ad Hoc Expert Committee, Rome, 22 March-2 April 1971. FAO Nutrition Meeting Report Series, no. 52; WHO Technical Report Series, no. 522. Rome: FAO and WHO.

_____. 1976a. Food and Nutrition Strategies in National Development. Ninth Report of the Joint FAO/WHO Expert Committee on Nutrition. Technical Report Series, no. 584. Geneva: World Health Organization.

Food and Agriculture Organization of the United Nations. Economic Commission for Africa. Women's Programme Unit. 1976b. The Role of Women in Population Dynamics Related to Food and Agriculture and Rural Development in Africa. Rome.

Forsyth, D. M. 1969. "A Longitudinal Study of Endemic Urinary Schistosomiasis in a Small East African Community." Bulletin of the World Health Organization 40: 771-83.

Fox, Greer Litton. 1973. "Some Determinants of Modernism Among Women in Ankara, Turkey." Journal of Marriage and the Family 35: 520-29.

Fox, R. H. 1953. "Energy Expenditure of Africans Engaged in Various Rural Activities." Ph.D. dissertation, University of London.

Foy, Henry and Nelson, George. 1963. "Helminths in the Etiology of Anemia in the Tropics, with Special Reference to Hookworms and Schistosomes." Parasitological Reviews 14: 240-62.

French, F. E. and Bierman, J. M. 1962. "Probabilities of Fetal

Mortality." Public Health Reports 77: 835-47.

Friedl, Ernestine, 1967. "The Position of Women: Appearance and Reality." Anthropological Quarterly 40: 97-108.

———. 1975. Women and Men: An Anthropologist's View. Basic Anthropology Units. New York: Holt, Rinehart & Winston.

Frisancho, A. Roberto. 1974. "Triceps Skinfold and Upper Arm Muscle Size Norms for Assessment of Nutritional Status." American Journal of Clinical Nutrition 27: 1052-58.

Frisch, Rose E. 1972. "Weight at Menarche: Similarity for Well-Nourished and Undernourished Girls at Differing Ages, and Evidence for Historical Constancy." Pediatrics 50: 445-50.

———. 1975. "Demographic Implications of the Biological Determinants of Female Fecundity." Social Biology 22: 17-22.

———. 1978a. "Nutrition, Fatness, and Fertility: The Effect of Food Intake on Reproductive Ability." In Nutrition and Human Reproduction, edited by W. Henry Mosley. New York: Plenum, pp. 91-122.

———. 1978b. "Population, Food Intake and Fertility." Science 199 (January 6): 22-30.

Frisch, Rose E. and McArthur, Janet W. 1974. "Menstrual Cycles: Fatness as a Determinant of Minimum Weight for Height Necessary for Their Maintenance or Onset." Science 184 (September 13): 949-51.

Gardner, Gerald W.; Edgerton, V. Reggie; Senewiratne, Brian; Barnard, R. James; and Ohira, Yoshinobu. 1977. "Physical Work Capacity and Metabolic Stress in Subjects with Iron-Deficiency Anemia." American Journal of Clinical Nutrition 30: 910-17.

Gavan, J. D. and Chandrasekara, I. S. 1979. The Impact of Public Foodgrain Distribution on Food Consumption and Welfare in Sri Lanka. Washington DC: International Food Policy Research Institute.

Geissler, Catherine; Calloway, Doris H.; and Margen, S. 1978. "Lactation and Pregnancy in Iran. II. Diet and Nutritional Status." American Journal of Clinical Nutrition 31: 341-54.

Giele, Janet Z. and Smock, Audrey C., eds. 1976. Woman: Roles and Status in Eight Countries. New York: Wiley.

Gilles, H. M.; Lawson, J. B.; Sibelas, M.; Voller, A.; and Allan, N. 1969. "Malaria, Anemia, and Pregnancy." Annals of Tropical Medicine and Parasitology 63: 245-63.

Golliday, Frederick. 1980. Health. Sector Policy Paper. 2nd ed. Washington, DC: International Bank for Reconstruction and Development.

Gopalan, C. 1958. "Studies on Lactation in Poor Indian Communities." Journal of Tropical Pediatrics 4: 87-97.

Gopaldas, Tara; Srinivasan, N.; Varadarajan, Indira; Shingwekar, Arvind G.; Seth, Ranja; Mathur, R. S.; and Bhargava, V. 1975. Project Poshak. 2 vols. New Delhi: CARE India.

Gray, Ronald H. 1979. "Biological Factors Other Than Nutrition and Lactation Which May Influence National Fertility: A Review." In Natural Fertility: Patterns and Determinants of Natural Fertility: Proceedings of a Seminar on Natural Fertility, edited by Henri Leridon and Jane A. Menken. Liege: Ordina Editions, pp. 217-51.

Greenfield, H. and Clark, J. A. 1974. "Energy Compensations Related to Child Bearing in Young Lufa Women." In Proceedings Xth Annual Symposium, Medical Society of Papua-New Guinea. Boroko, New Guinea.

Greenham, R. 1978. "Anaemia and Schistosoma Haematobium Infection in the North-Eastern Province of Kenya." Transactions of the Royal Society of Tropical Medicine and Hygiene 72: 72-75.

Gross, Daniel R. and Underwood, Barbara A. 1971. "Technological Change and Caloric Costs: Sisal Agriculture in Northeastern Brazil." American Anthropologist 73: 725-40.

Gueri, Miguel; Jutsum, Peter; and Sorhaindo, Bernard. 1982.

"Anthropometric Assessment of Nutritional Status in Pregnant Women: A Reference Table of Weight-for-Height by Week of Pregnancy." American Journal of Clinical Nutrition 35: 609-11.

Guillebaud, John; Bonnar, John; Morehead, Jean; and Matthews, Anne. 1976. "Menstrual Blood-Loss with Intrauterine Devices." Lancet 1 (February 21): 387-90.

Gulick, John and Gulick, Margaret E. 1974. "Varieties of Domestic Social Organization in the Iranian City of Isfahan." New York Academy of Sciences/Annals of the Lyceum of Natural History of New York 220: 441-69.

Gupta, R. and Sharma, I. 1980. "An Overview of the Dietary Consumption Pattern of Pregnant and Lactating Mothers of Haryana Region, Hissar." Indian Journal of Nutrition and Dietetics 17: 13-19.

Guyer, Jane I. 1980. "Household Budgets and Women's Incomes." Working Paper, no. 28. Brookline, MA: African Studies Center, Boston University.

Gwatkin, D. C.; Wilcox, J. R.; and Wray, Joe D. 1980. "The Policy Implications of Field Experiments in Primary Health and Nutrition Care." Social Science and Medicine 14C: 121-28.

Habicht, Jean-Pierre; Yarbrough, Charles; Lechtig, Aaron; and Klein, Robert E. 1973. "Relationships of Birthweight, Maternal Nutrition and Infant Mortality." Nutrition Reports International 7: 533-46.

Haddad, Wadi D. 1980. Education. Sector Policy Paper. Washington, DC: International Bank for Reconstruction and Development.

Hammond, Dorothy and Jablow, Alta. 1976. Women in Cultures of the World. Cummings Modular Program in Anthropology. Menlo Park, CA: Cummings.

Hardy, Janet B. and Mellits, E. David. 1977. "Relationship of Low Birth Weight to Maternal Characteristics of Age, Parity, Education and Body Size." In The Epidemiology of Prematurity, edited by Dwayne M. Reed and Fiona J. Stanley. Baltimore: Urban & Schwarzenberg.

Harlap, Susan; Prywes, Rachel; Grover, Norman B.; and Davies, A. Michael. 1977. "Maternal, Perinatal and Infant Health in Bedouin and Jews in Southern Israel." Israel Journal of Medical Sciences 13: 514-28.

Harrison, G. A.; Boyce, A. J.; Platt, C. M.; and Sejeantson, S. 1975. "Body Composition Changes during Lactation in a New Guinea Population." Annals of Human Biology 2: 395-98.

Hart, Gillian. 1975. "Women's Participation in the Labor Force: Implications for Employment and Health/Nutrition Programs." [Ithaca, NY: Department of Agricultural Economics, Cornell University.]

Hauck, Hazel M. 1963. "Weight Changes During Pregnancy, Awo Omamma, Nigeria, 1960." Journal of Obstetrics and Gynaecology of the British Commonwealth 70: 885-90.

Hegsted, D. M. 1974. "Energy Needs and Energy Utilization." Nutrition Reviews 32: 33-38.

Heimendinger, Jerianne; Zeitlin, Marian F.; and Austin, James E. 1981. Nutrition Intervention in Developing Countries. Vol. 3. Study IV: Formulated Foods. Cambridge, MA: Oelgeschlager, Gunn & Hain.

Heller, Peter S. and Drake, William D. 1979. "Malnutrition, Child Morbidity and the Family Decision Process." Journal of Development Economics 6: 203-35.

Hendricks, Charles H. and Brenner, William E. 1971. "Toxemia of Pregnancy: Relationship Between Fetal Weight, Fetal Survival, and the Maternal State." American Journal of Obstetrics and Gynecology 109: 225-33.

Herrin, Alejandro N. 1979. "Rural Electrification and Fertility Change in the Southern Philippines." Population and Development Review 5: 61-86.

Higgins, Agnes. 1972. "Montreal Diet Dispensary Study in Nutritional

Supplementation and the Outcome of Pregnancy." Washington, DC: National Academy of Sciences.

Hijazi, Saad S. 1977. Child Growth and Nutrition in Jordan. Amman: Royal Scientific Society Press.

Hillman, Robert W.; Slater, Paul; and Nelson, Marjory J. 1970. "Season of Birth, Parental Age, Menarcheal Age and Body Form: Some Interrelationships in Young Women." Human Biology 42: 570-80.

Ho, Teresa J. 1979. "Time Costs of Child Rearing in the Rural Philippines." Population and Development Review 5: 643-62.

Hollinsteiner, Mary R. 1978. "Peri-urban Malnutrition, a Neglected Problem: Patterns and Approaches." Carnets de l'enfance 43 (July/September): 25-46.

Horowitz, Grace. 1980. "Distribution of Food and Other Resources Within the Family in the Third World." Report to the Nutrition Economics Group, Office of Nutrition Development Support Bureau. Washington, DC: U.S. Agency for International Development.

Hoskins, Marilyn W. 1979. "Women in Forestry for Local Community Development: A Programming Guide." Washington, DC: Office of Women in Development, U.S. Agency for International Development.

Howie, P. W.; McNeilly, A. S.; Houston, M. J.: Cook, A.; and Boyle, H. 1982. "Fertility after Childbirth: Postpartum Ovulation and Menstruation in Bottle and Breast-Feeding Mothers." Journal of Clinical Endocrinology 17: 323-32.

Huffman, Sandra L. 1982. "Influencing Natural Fertility in Developing Countries." Paper prepared for the National Academy of Sciences, Committee on Population and Demography Conference on Fertility Research and Population in Developing Countries, Washington, DC, November 22-23.

Huffman, Sandra L.; Chowdhury, A. K. M. Alauddin; and Mosley, W. Henry. 1978a. "Postpartum Amenorrhea: How Is It Affected by Maternal Nutritional Status?" Science 200 (June 9): 1155-57.

Huffman, Sandra L.; Chowdhury, A. K. M. Alauddin; Chakraborty, J.; and Simpson, Nancy K. 1980a. "Breast-Feeding Patterns in Rural Bangladesh." American Journal of Clinical Nutrition 33: 144-54.

Huffman, Sandra L.; Chowdhury, A. K. M. Alauddin; and Sykes, Zenas M. 1980b. "Lactation and Fertility in Rural Bangladesh." Population Studies 34: 337-47.

Huffman, Sandra L.; Chowdhury, A. K. M. Alauddin; Chakraborty, J.; and Mosley, W. Henry. 1978b. "Nutrition and Post-Partum Amenorrhea in Rural Bangladesh." Population Studies 32: 251-60.

Hunter, John Melton. 1967. "Seasonal Hunger in a Part of the West African Savanna: A Survey of Bodyweights in Nangodi, North-East Ghana." Institute of British Geographers Transactions and Papers 41: 167-85.

Hytten, Frank E. and Leitch, Isabella. 1971. The Physiology of Human Pregnancy. 2nd ed. Oxford, England: Blackwell; Philadelphia: Lippincott.

ICRW. See International Center for Research on Women.

Immink, Maarten D. C.; Sanjur, Diva; and Colon, Mirta. 1981. "Home Gardens and the Energy and Nutrient Intakes of Women and Preschoolers in Rural Puerto Rico." Ecology of Food and Nutrition 11: 191-99.

Ingalls, Theodore Hunt; Draper, Ruth; and Teel, Harold M. 1938. "Vitamin C in Human Pregnancy and Lactation." American Journal of Diseases of Children 56: 1011-19.

Insull, W., Jr.; Hirsch, J.; James, T.; and Ahrens, E. H., Jr. 1959. "The Fatty Acids in Human Milk. II. Alteration Produced by Manipulation of Caloric Balance and Exchange of Dietary Fats." Journal of Clinical Investigations 38: 443-50.

International Center for Research on Women. 1980. The Productivity of Women in Developing Countries: Measurement Issues and Recommendations. Washington, DC: The Office of Women in Development,

U.S. Agency for International Development.

International Labour Office. 1978. Yearbook of Labour Statistics 1978. Geneva.

Jacobson, Doranne. 1978. "The Chaste Wife: Cultural Norm and Individual Experience." In American Studies of the Anthropology of India, edited by Sylvia Vatuk. New Delhi: Manohar Press under the auspices of the American Institute of Indian Studies, pp. 95-138.

Jansen, A. A. J.; Lakhani, S. A.; 't Mannetje, W.; and Kusin, Jane A. 1980. "Some Nutritional Aspects of Pregnancy in Rural Kenya." The East African Medical Journal 57: 97-104.

Jansen, G. R.; Jansen, N. B.; Shigetomi, C. T.; and Harper, J. M. 1977. "Effect of Income and Geographical Region on the Nutritional Value of Diets in Brazil." American Journal of Clinical Nutrition 30: 955-64.

Jaszmann, L.; VanLith, N. D.; and Zaat, J. C. 1979. "The Age of Menopause in the Netherlands." International Journal of Fertility 14: 106.

Jathar, V. S.; Kamath, S. A.; Parikh, M. N.; Rege, D. V.; and Satoskar, R. S. 1970. "Maternal Milk and Serum Vitamin B12, Folic Acid, and Protein Levels in Indian Subjects." Archives of Diseases in Childhood 45: 236-41.

Javillonar, Gloria; Zivetz, Laurie; Thompson, Susan; and Griffith, Janet. 1979. Rural Development, Women's Role, and Fertility in Developing Countries: Review of the Literature. [Research Triangle Park, NC]: Research Triangle Institute and South East Consortium for International Development.

Jayme-Ho, Teresa. 1976. "Time Allocation, Home Production and Labor Force Participation of Married Women: An Exploratory Survey." Institute of Economic Development and Research Discussion Paper, no. 76-8. [Dillman, Quezon City]: University of the Philippines.

Jelliffe, Derrick Brian and Jelliffe, E. F. Patrice. 1967. "Parallel Food Classifications in Developing and Industrialized Countries." American Journal of Clinical Nutrition 20: 279-81.

_____ 1978. Human Milk in the Modern World: Psychosocial, Nutritional and Economic Significance. London: Oxford University Press.

_____ 1981. "Appropriate Technology and Nutritional Assessment." In Advances in International Maternal and Child Health, vol. 1, edited by Derrick Brian Jelliffe and E. F. Patrice Jelliffe. New York: Oxford University Press.

Jelliffe, Derrick Brian and Maddocks, I. 1964. "Notes on Ecologic Malnutrition in the New Guinea Highlands." Clinical Pediatrics 3: 432-38.

Jiminez, Marcia Houdek and Newton, Niles. 1979. "Activity and Work During Pregnancy and the Postpartum Period: A Cross-Cultural Study of 202 Societies." American Journal of Obstetrics and Gynecology 135: 171-76.

Johnson, Bruce F. and Meyer, Anthony J. 1977. "Nutrition, Health, and Population in Strategies for Rural Development." Economic Development and Cultural Change 26: 1-23.

Johnston, Francis E. 1974. "Control of Age at Menarche." Human Biology 46: 159-71.

Jones, Edna M. and Munger, Sara J. 1978. Applications of a Field Guide for Evaluation of Nutrition Education to Programs in the Philippines. Allison Park, PA: Synectics Corp.

Jordan, Peter and Webbe, Gerald. 1969. Human Schistosomiasis. London: Heinemann Medical.

Karmarkar, M. G.; Kapur, J.; Deodhar, A. D.; and Ramakrishnan, C. V. 1959. "Diet Survey of Lactating Women in Different Socio Economic Groups and the Effects of Socio Economic Status and Stage of Lactation on the Proximate Principles and Essential Amino Acids of Human Milk." Indian Journal of Medical Research 62: 571-76.

Karyadi, Darwin and Basta, Samir S. 1973. "Nutrition and Health of

Indonesian Construction Workers: Endurance Anemia." Staff Working Paper, no. 152. Washington, DC: Research Division, Transportation Department, International Bank for Reconstruction and Development.

Kassoudji, S. and Mueller, Eva. 1980. The Economic and Demographic Status of Female Headed Households in Botswana. Ann Arbor: Population Studies Center, University of Michigan.

Katona-Apte, Judit. 1975. "The Relevance of Nourishment to the Reproductive Cycle of the Female in India." In Being Female: Reproduction, Power, and Change, edited by Dana Raphael. Mouton World Anthropology Series. The Hague: Mouton, pp. 43-48.

_____ 1977a. "The Socio-Cultural Aspects of Food Avoidance in a Low-Income Population in Tamilnad, South India." Journal of Tropical Pediatrics and Environmental Child Health 23: 83-90.

_____ 1977b. "Urbanization, Income and Sociocultural Factors Relevant to Nutrition in Tamil Nadu." Social Action 27: 266-78.

Kawata, Kazayoshi. 1978. "Water and Other Environmental Interventions-- The Minimum Investment Concept." American Journal of Clinical Nutrition 31: 2114-23.

Keeping, J. D.; Chang, A.; Morrison, J.; and Esler, E. J. 1979. "Birth Weight: Analysis of Variance and the Linear Additive Model." British Journal of Obstetrics and Gynaecology 86: 437-42.

Kelly, F. C. and Snedden, W. W. 1960. Endemic Goitre. WHO Monograph Series, no. 44. Geneva.

Kelly, Sally; Hook, Ernest B.; Janerich, Dwight T.; and Porter, Ian H., eds. 1976. Birth Defects: Risks and Consequences. Proceedings of a Conference Held in Albany, New York, November 1974. Birth Defects Institute Symposia. New York: Academic Press.

Kendall, Katherine Wakeman. 1968. "Personality Development in an Iranian Village: An Analysis of Socialization Practices and the Development of the Woman's Role." Ph.D. dissertation, University of Washington.

Kennedy, Elaine T.; Gershoff, Stanley; Reed, R.; and Austin, James E. 1979. "Effects of WIC Supplemental Feeding on Birth Weight." Cambridge, MA: Department of Nutrition, Harvard University.

Keusch, Gerald T. 1972. "Subclinical Malabsorption in Thailand. I. Intestinal Absorption in Thai Children." American Journal of Clinical Nutrition 25: 1062-66.

Keys, Ancel Benjamin; Brovek, Josef; Henschel, Austin; Mickelsen, Olaf; and Taylor, Henry Longstreet. 1950. The Biology of Human Starvation. 2 vols. Minneapolis: University of Minnesota Press.

Kielmann, Arnfried A.; Taylor, Carl E.; and Parker, Robert L. 1978. "The Narangwal Nutrition Study: A Summary Review." American Journal of Clinical Nutrition 31: 2040-52.

Knodel, John. 1977. "Breast-Feeding and Population Growth." Science 198 (December 16): 1111-15.

Kon, Stanislaw Kazimierz and Mawson, E. H. 1950. "Human Milk." Special Reports Series, no. 219. London: Medical Research Council.

Korean Statistical Association. 1977. Food and Nutrient Intake Studies of Rural Population in Korea. Seoul.

Kortmann, Henricus Franciscus Constantinius Maria. 1972. Malaria and Pregnancy. Utrecht: Drukkerij Elinkwijk.

Kraut, H. A. and Muller, E. A. 1946. "Caloric Intake and Industrial Output." Science 104 (November 29): 495-97.

KSA. See Korean Statistical Association.

Kusin, Jane A.; Kardjati, Sri; de With, C.; and Sudibia, Ig. K. 1979. "Nutrition and Nutritional Status of Rural Women in East Java." Tropical and Geographical Medicine 31: 571-85.

Kusin, Jane A.; Kardjati, Sri; Suryohudoyo, Porind; and de With, C. 1980. "Anemia and Hypovitaminosis A Among Rural Women in East Java,

Indonesia." Tropical and Geographical Medicine 32: 30-39.

Lapham, Robert J. and Von Wie, William A. 1976. "Maternal and Child Health and Family Planning Projects in Remote Rural Areas of Four Countries." Paper presented to the Annual Meeting of the American Public Health Association, Miami, October 17-21.

Latham, Michael C. 1975. "Nutrition and Infection in National Development." Science 188 (May 9): 561-65.

Latham, Michael C. and Brooks, Mark. 1977. "The Relationship of Nutrition and Health to Worker Productivity in Kenya." Technical Memorandum, no. 26. Washington, DC: Transportation Department, International Bank for Reconstruction and Development.

Lechtig, Aaron and Arroyave, Guillermo. 1977. "The Nutrition Problem in Latin America: Definition, Causes, and Remedial Actions." Bulletin of the Pan American Health Organization 11: 319-31.

Lechtig, Aaron; Delgado, Hernán; Lasky, Robert E.; Yarbrough, Charles; Martorell, Reynaldo; Habicht, Jean-Pierre; and Klein, Robert E. 1975a. "Effect of Improved Nutrition During Pregnancy and Lactation on Developmental Retardation and Infant Mortality." In Proceedings of the Western Hemisphere Nutrition Congress IV, 1974, edited by Philip L. White and Nancy Selvey. Chicago: American Medical Association, pp. 117-25.

Lechtig, Aaron; Delgado, Hernán; Lasky, Robert E.; Yarbrough, Charles; Klein, Robert E.; Habicht, Jean-Pierre; and Behar, Moisés. 1975b. "Maternal Nutrition and Fetal Growth in Developing Countries." American Journal of Diseases of Children 129: 553-56.

Lechtig, Aaron; Delgado, Hernán; Martorell, Reynaldo; Richardson, Douglas; Yarbrough, Charles; and Klein, Robert E. 1978a. "Effect of Maternal Nutrition on Infant Mortality." In Nutrition and Human Reproduction, edited by W. Henry Mosley. New York: Plenum, pp. 147-74.

Lechtig, Aaron; Delgado, Hernán; Martorell, Reynaldo; Yarbrough, Charles; and Klein, Robert E. 1978b. "Effect of Food Supplementation on Blood Pressure and on the Prevalence of Edema and Proteinuria During Pregnancy." Journal of Tropical Pediatrics and Environmental Child Health 24: 70-76.

_____ 1979. "Maternofetal Nutrition." In Human Nutrition: A Comprehensive Treatise. Vol. 2, Nutrition and Growth, edited by Derrick Brian Jelliffe and E. F. Patrice Jelliffe. New York: Plenum, pp. 79-127.

Lechtig, Aaron; Habicht, Jean-Pierre; Delgado, Hernán; Klein, Robert E.; Yarbrough, Charles; and Martorell, Reynaldo. 1975c. "Effect of Food Supplementation During Pregnancy on Birthweight." Pediatrics 56: 508-20.

Lechtig, Aaron; Klein, Robert E.; Daza, Carlos Hernán; Read, Merrill S.; and Kahn, Samuel G. 1982. "Effects of Maternal Nutrition on Infant Health: Implications for Action." Journal of Tropical Pediatrics 28: 273-86.

Leslie, Joanne. 1977. "The Use of Mass Media in Health Education Campaigns." Educational Broadcasting International 11: 136-142.

LeVine, Robert A. 1980. "Influences of Women's Schooling on Maternal Behavior in the Third World." Comparative Education Review 24 (no. 2, pt. 2): S78-105.

Levinson, F. James. 1974. Morinda: An Economic Analysis of Malnutrition Among Young Children in Rural India. Cambridge, MA: Cornell/MIT International Nutrition Policy Series.

Lindblad, B.A. and Rahimtoola, Razia J. 1974. "A Pilot Study of the Quality of Human Milk in a Lower Socio-Economic Group in Karachi, Pakistan." Acta Paediatrica Scandinavica 63: 125-28.

Lindblad, B. S.; Ljunggrust, A.; Gebre-Medhun, M.; and Rahimtoola, Razia J. 1977. "The Composition and Yield of Human Milk in Developing Countries." In Food and Immunology. Symposium on Food and Immunology, edited by Leif Hambraeus. Stockholm: Almqvist & Wiksell.

Lockheed, Marlaine E.; Jameson, Dean T.; and Lau, Lawrence J. 1980.

"Farmer Education and Farm Efficiency: A Summary." Economic Development and Cultural Change 29 (October): 37-76.

Longhurst, Richard and Payne, Philip. 1979. "Seasonal Aspects of Nutrition: Review of Evidence and Policy Implications." Discussion Paper, no. 145. Brighton, England: Institute of Development Studies, University of Sussex.

Lunn, P. G.; Prentice, A. M.; Austin, S.; and Whithead, Roger G. 1980. "Influence of Maternal Diet on Plasma-Prolactin Levels During Lactation." Lancet 1 (March 22): 623-25.

McCann, Margaret F.; Liskin, Laurie S.; Piotrow, Phyllis T.; Rinehart, Ward; and Fox, Gordon. 1981. "Breast-Feeding, Fertility and Family Planning." Population Reports, Ser. J. no. 24.

McDonald, Elaine C.; Hsueh, Andie M.; and Sherwin, Roger. c.1980. "The Bacon Chow Study: Maternal Nutritional Supplementation and Birth Weight of Offspring." Houston: School of Public Health, University of Texas.

McDonald, Maurice E. 1977. Food, Stamps, and Income Maintenance. Institute for Research on Poverty Policy Analysis Series. New York: Academic Press.

McGill, Henry C., Jr. 1979. "Appraisal of Cholesterol as a Causative Factor in Artherogenesis." American Journal of Clinical Nutrition 32: 2632-36.

Macgregor, J. D. and Avery J. G. 1974. "Malaria Transmission and Fetal Growth." British Medical Journal 3 (August 17): 433-36.

McGuire, Judith Snavely. 1979. "Seasonal Changes in Energy Expenditure and Work Patterns of Rural Guatemalan Women." Ph.D. dissertation, Massachusetts Institute of Technology.

McKinlay, Sonja; Jefferys, Margot; and Thompson, Barbara. 1972. "An Investigation of the Age at Menopause." Journal of Biosocial Science 41: 161-73.

MacMahon, Brian and Worcester, Jane. 1966. "Age at Menopause: United States--1960-62." Vital and Health Statistics, Ser. 11: Data from the National Health Survey, no. 19. Public Health Service Publication no. 1000-Ser. 11- no. 19. Washington, DC: Public Health Service, U.S. Department of Health, Education, and Welfare.

McSweeney, Brenda Gael and Freedman, Marion. 1980. "Lack of Time as an Obstacle to Women's Education: The Case of Upper Volta." Comparative Education Review 24 (no. 2, pt. 2): S124-39.

Madhaven, S. 1965. "Age of Menarche of South Indian Girls Belonging to the States of Madras and Kerala." Indian Journal of Medical Research 53: 669-73.

Magnarella, Paul J. 1974. Tradition and Change in a Turkish Town. New York: Halsted.

Makhlouf, Carla and Overmeyer, Gerald J. 1978. "Women and Social Change in Urban North Yemen." In Women's Status and Fertility in the Muslim World, edited by James Allman. New York: Praeger, pp. 333-47.

Martin, F. I. R.; Wyatt, G. B.; Griew, A. R.; Haurahelia, Mary; and Higginbotham, Linda. 1980. "Diabetes Mellitus in Urban and Rural Communities in Papua New Guinea." Diabetologia 18: 369-74.

Martínez, Celia; Madrigal, Herlinda; Gonzalez, Olga; and Garcia, Susana. 1977. "Modificaciones dieteticas en las muyeres embarazadas y lactantes del medio rural." Cuadernos de Nutricion 2: 83-89.

Massey, Linda K. and Davison, Meredith A. 1979. "Effect of Oral Contraceptives on Nutritional Status." American Family Physician 19: 119-23.

Mata, Leonardo J. 1978. The Children of Santa María Cauqué: A Prospective Field Study of Health and Growth. International Nutrition Policy Series. Cambridge, MA: MIT Press.

Matsuo, Takefumi. 1967. "Hypertension in Indonesia." Kobe Journal of Medical Science 13: 171-79.

Mehrotra, M. L.; Gautam, K. D.; Pande, D. C.; Chaube, C. K.; Dixit, R.; Malhotra, A.; and Kushwaha, S. 1974. "Compatibility of Oral Contraceptive with Anti-Tubercular Chemotherapy in Female Pulmonary Tuberculosis Patients." Indian Journal of Medical Research 62: 1782-86.

Menken, Jane A. and Bongaarts, John. 1978. "Reproductive Models in the Study of Nutrition-Fertility Interrelationships." In Nutrition and Human Reproduction, edited by W. Henry Mosley. New York: Plenum, pp. 261-312.

Menken, Jane A.; Trussell, James; and Watkins, Susan. 1981. "The Nutrition Fertility Link: An Evaluation of the Evidence." Journal of Interdisciplinary History 11: 425-41.

Mernissi, Fatima. 1978. "The Patriarch in the Moroccan Family: Myth or Reality?" In Women's Status and Fertility in the Muslim World, edited by James Allman. New York: Praeger, pp. 312-32.

Merrick, Thomas William and Schmink, Marianne. 1983. "Households Headed by Women and Urban Poverty in Brazil." In Women and Poverty in the Third World, edited by Mayra Buvinić, Margaret A. Lycette, and William Paul McGreevey. Baltimore: Johns Hopkins University Press, pp. 244-71.

Metcoff, Jack; Costiloe, P.; Crosby, W. M.; Bentle, L.; Dutta, Seshuchalam; Sandstead, Harold H.; Bodwell, C. D.; Weaver, F.; and McClain, P. E. [1979] "Maternal Nutrition and Fetal Outcome." In Nutrition of the Child: Maternal Nutritional Status and Fetal Outcome. Vol. I. [Houston]: Children's Nutrition Research Center, Department of Pediatrics, Baylor College of Medicine and Texas Children's Hospital.

Miall, W. E.; Kass, E. H.; Ling, J.; and Stuart, K. L. 1962. "Factors Influencing Arterial Pressure in the General Population in Jamaica." British Medical Journal 2 (August 25): 497-506.

Micklewait, Donald R.; Riegelman, Mary Ann; and Sweet, Charles F. 1976. Women in Rural Development: A Survey of Women in Ghana, Lesotho, Kenya, Nigeria, Bolivia, Paraguay, and Peru. Boulder, CO: Westview Press.

Miller, D. S. 1979. "Prevalence of Nutritional Problems in the World." Proceedings of the Nutrition Society 38: 197-205.

Miller, David C.; Nichaman, Milton Z.; and Lane, J. Michael. 1977. "Simplified Field Assessment of Nutritional Status in Early Childhood: Practical Suggestions for Developing Countries." Bulletin of the World Health Organization 55: 79-86.

Miller, G. H. and Hughes, L. R. 1970. "Lactation and Genital Involution Effects of a New Low-Dose Oral Contraceptive on Breast-feeding Mothers and Their Infants." Obstetrics and Gynecology 35: 44-50.

Mirrlees, J. A. 1975. "A Pure Theory of Under-developed Economies Using a Relationship Between Consumption and Production." New Haven, CT: Economic Growth Center, Yale University.

Montgomery, Edward. 1978. "Towards Representative Energy Data: The Machiguenga Study." Federation Proceedings 37: 61-64.

Montgomery, Edward and Johnson, Allen. 1977. "Machiguenga Energy Expenditure." Ecology of Food and Nutrition 6: 97-105.

Mora, J. O.; de Paredes, B.; Wagner, M.; de Navarro, L.; Suescun, J.; Christiansen, Niels; and Herrera, M. G. 1979. "Nutrition Supplementation and the Outcome of Pregnancy. I. Birth Weight." American Journal of Clinical Nutrition 32: 455-62.

Morley, David; Woodland, Margaret; and Cuthbertson, W. F. J. 1964. "Controlled Trial of Pyrimethamaine in Pregnant Women in an African Village." British Medical Journal 1 (March 14): 667-68.

Mosley, W. Henry. 1979. "The Effects of Nutrition on Natural Fertility." In Natural Fertility: Patterns and Determinants of Natural Fertility: Proceedings of a Seminar on Natural Fertility, edited by Henri Leridon and Jane A. Menken. Liege, Belgium: Ordina Editions, pp. 83-105.

Mott, K. 1980. "Schistosomiasis." Paper presented to the Workshop on the Development of Guidelines to Assess the Social and Economic Consequences of the Tropical Diseases, Geneva, October 22-27.

Mueller, Eva. 1979. "Household Structure, Time Use, and Income Distribution in Rural Botswana." Paper presented to the Annual Meeting of the Population Association of America, Philadelphia, April 27.

Muller, R. 1981. "Guinea-Worm Infection." In Seasonal Dimensions to Rural Poverty, edited by Robert Chambers, Richard Longhurst, and Arnold Pacey. London: Pinter; Totowa, NJ: Allanheld, Osmun, pp. 125-27.

Murray, M. J.; Murray, Anne B.; Murray, Megan B.; and Murray, N.J. 1978. "The Adverse Effect of Iron Repletion on the Course of Certain Infections." British Medical Journal 2 (6145): 1113-15.

Naeye, Richard L.; Blanc, William A.; and Paul, Cheryl. 1973. "Effects of Maternal Nutrition on the Human Fetus." Pediatrics 52: 494-503.

National Institute of Nutrition. 1980. Annual Report, January 1, 1979 to December 31, 1979. Hyderabad: Indian Council of Medical Research.

National Research Council. Committee on Maternal Nutrition. 1970. Maternal Nutrition and the Course of Pregnancy: Summary Report. Washington, DC: National Academy of Sciences.

Natonal Research Council, Food and Nutrition Board. 1980. Recommended Dietary Allowances. Washington, DC: National Academy of Sciences.

Newton, John. 1972. "Secondary Amenorrhea, Oligomenorrhea, and Anovular Menstrual Cycles." British Journal of Hospital Medicine 7: 564-72.

NIN. See National Institute of Nutrition.

Niswander, Kenneth R. 1977. "Obstetric Factors Related to Prematurity." In The Epidemiology of Prematurity, edited by Dwayne M. Reed and Fiona J. Stanley. Baltimore: Urban & Schwarzenberg, pp. 249-68.

Noel, Gordon L.; Suh, Han K.; and Frantz, Andrew G. 1974. "Prolactin Release During Nursing and Breast Stimulation in Postpartum and Nonpostpartum Subjects." Journal of Clinical Endocrinology and Metabolism 38: 413-23.

Noguer, A. 1980. "Malaria." Paper presented to the Workshop on the Development of Guidelines to Assess the Social and Economic Consequences of the Tropical Diseases, Geneva, October 22-27.

Norgan, N. G.; Ferro-Luzzi, A.; and Durnin, John Valentine George Andrew. 1974. "The Energy and Nutrient Intake and Energy Expenditure of 204 New Guinean Adults." Philosophical Transactions of the Royal Society of London 268B: 309-48.

NRC. See National Research Council.

Nutrition Foundation of the Philippines, Field Service Section. 1977. "Dietary Survey among Pregnant and Lactating Women in a Resettlement. 2. Twenty-Four-Hour-Recall." Philippine Journal of Nutrition 30: 119-22.

Odutan, S. Olu and Ayeni, O. 1974. "Correlates of Low Birth Weights in Two Nigerian Communities." Tropical and Geographical Medicine 28: 220-23.

Okediji, Francis Oluokon. 1975. "Socioeconomic Status and Attitudes to Public Health Problems in the Western Seate: A Case Study of Ibadan." In Population Growth and Social-Economic Change in West Africa, edited by John C. Caldwell. New York: Columbia University Press, pp. 275-97.

O'Laughlin, Bridget. 1974. "Mediation of Contradiction: Why Mbum Women Do Not Eat Chicken." In Woman, Culture and Society, edited by Michelle Zimbalist Rosaldo and Louise Lamphere. Stanford, CA: Stanford University Press, pp. 301-18.

Operations Research Group. 1979. "Food Habits Survey--Gujarat and Maharashtra." Conducted for the Protein Food Association of India. New Delhi.

Oppong, Christine. 1980. "A Synopsis of Seven Roles and Statuses of Women." Population and Labour Policies Programme Working Paper, no. 94. Geneva: International Labour Organization.

Oshima, Harry T. 1967. "Food Consumption, Nutrition, and Economic Development in Asian Countries." Economic Development and Cultural

Change 15: 385-97.

———. 1971. "Seasonality and Underemployment in Monsoon Asia." Philippine Economics Journal 10: 63-97.

Osteria, Trinidad S. 1978. "Variations on Fertility with Breast-feeding and Contraception in Urban Filipino Women: Implications for a Nutrition Program." In Nutrition and Human Reproduction, edited by W. Henry Mosley. New York: Plenum, pp. 411-32.

Page, Lot B.; Damon, Albert; and Moellering, Robert C., Jr. 1974. "Antecedents of Cardiovascular Disease in Six Solomon Island Societies." Circulation 49: 1132-46.

Pala, Achola Okeyo. 1979. "Women in the Household Economy: Managing Multiple Roles." Studies in Family Planning 10: 337-43.

Palmer, Ingrid. 1981. "Seasonal Dimensions of Women's Roles." In Seasonal Dimensions to Rural Poverty, edited by Robert Chambers, Richard Longhurst, and Arnold Pacey. London: Pinter; Totowa, NJ: Allanheld, Osmun, pp. 195-201.

———. 1979. "The Nemow Case: Case Studies on the Impact of Large Scale Development Projects on Women: A Series for Planners." Working Paper no. 7. New York: The Population Council.

———. 1980. "Women in Rural Development." International Development Review 22 (2-3): 39-45.

Papanek, Hanna. 1973. "Purdah: Separate Worlds and Symbolic Shelter." Comparative Studies in Society and History 14: 289-325.

Papda, T. S. 1980. Sex Discrimination in the Urban Labour Market: Some Propositions Based on Indian Evidence. Geneva: International Labour Office.

Parker, Seymour and Parker, Hilda. 1979. "The Myth of Male Superiority: Rise and Demise." American Anthropologist 81: 289-309.

Parischa, Swaran. 1958. "A Survey of Dietary Intake in a Group of Poor, Pregnant and Lactating Women." Indian Journal of Medical Research 46: 605-09.

Passmore, Reginald; Nichol, B. M.; and Rao, M. Narayana in collaboration with Beaton, George H. and Bengoa, J. M. 1974. Handbook of Human Nutritional Requirements. WHO Monograph Series, no. 61. Geneva: World Health Organization.

Paul, Alison A.; Müller, Elisabeth M.; and Whitehead, Roger G. 1979a. "The Quantitative Effects of Maternal Dietary Energy Intake on Pregnancy and Lactation in Rural Gambian Women." Transactions of the Royal Society of Tropical Medicine and Hygiene 73: 686-92.

———. 1979b. "Seasonal Variations in Energy Intake, Body-Weight and Skinfold Thickness in Pregnant and Lactating Women in Rural Gambia." Proceedings of the Nutrition Society 38 (2): 28A.

Paul, Lois. 1974. "The Mastery of Work and the Mystery of Sex in a Guatemalan Village." In Woman, Culture and Society, edited by Michelle Zimbalist Rosaldo and Louise Lamphere. Stanford, CA: Stanford University Press, pp. 281-99.

Perez, Alfredo; Vela, Patricio; Potter, Robert G.; and Masnick, George S. 1971. "Timing and Sequence of Resuming Ovulation and Menstruation After Childbirth." Population Studies 25: 491-503.

Peters, Wallace and Gilles, H. M. 1977. A Colour Atlas of Tropical Medicine and Parasitology. London: Wolfe Medical Publications.

Picone, Thomas A.; Allen, Lindsay H.; Olsen, Pauline, N.; and Ferris, Margaret E. 1982. "Pregnancy Outcomes in North American Women. II. Effects of Diet, Cigarette Smoking, Stress and Weight Gain on Placentas and on Neonatal Physical and Behavioral Characteristics." American Journal of Clinical Nutrition 36: 121-24.

Pinstrup-Andersen, Per; de Londoño, Norha Ruiz; and Hoover, Edward. 1976. "The Impact of Increasing Food Supply on Human Nutrition: Implications for Commodity Priorities in Agricultural Research and Policy."

American Journal of Agricultural Economics 58: 131-42.

Pitkin, Roy M. 1979. "Assessment of Nutritional Status of Mother, Fetus, and Newborn." In Nutrition of the Child: Maternal Nutritional Status and Fetal Outcome. Vol. 1. [Houston]: Children's Nutrition Research Center, Department of Pediatrics, Baylor College of Medicine and Texas Children's Hospital.

Popkin, Barry M. 1978. "Nutrition and Labor Productivity." Social Science and Medicine 12: 117-25.

_____. 1981. "Community-Level Considerations in Nutrition Planning in Low Income Nations." Ecology of Food and Nutrition 10: 227-36.

Popkin, Barry M. and Latham, Michael C. 1973. "The Limitations and Dangers of Commerciogenic Nutritious Foods." American Journal of Clinical Nutrition 26: 1015-23.

Popkin, Barry M. and Solon, Florentino S. 1976. "Income, Time, the Working Mother and Child Nutriture." Journal of Tropical Pediatrics and Environmental Child Health 22: 156-66.

Popkin, Barry M.; Akin, John; Haines, Pamela; McDonald, Maurice; and Spicer, Deborah. 1980. Nutrition Program Options for Maternal and Child Health. Special Report Series, no. SR 28. Madison: Institute for Research on Poverty, University of Wisconsin-Madison.

Porter, Michael J. 1981. "Infectious Skin Diseases." In Seasonal Dimensions to Rural Poverty, edited by Robert Chambers, Richard Longhurst, and Arnold Pacey. London: Pinter; Totowa, NJ: Allanheld, Osmun, pp. 114-16.

Potter, Robert G.; Wyon, John B.; New, M. L.; and Gordon, John E. 1965. "Fetal Wastage in Eleven Punjab Villages." Human Biology 37: 262-73.

Prasad, Ananda S.; Moghissi, Kamran S.; Lee, Kai Y.; Oberleas, Donald; and Stryker, Joan C. 1977. "Effect of Oral Contraceptives on Micronutrients and Changes in Trace Elements Due to Pregnancy." In Nutritional Impacts on Women Throughout Life with Emphasis on Reproduction, edited by Kamran S. Moghissi and Tommy N. Evans. Hagerstown, MD: Harper & Row, pp. 160-88.

Prema, K.; Naidu, A. N.; Neelakumari, S.; and Ramalakshmi, B. A. 1981. "Nutrition-Fertility Interaction in Lactating Women of Low Income Groups." British Journal of Nutrition 45: 461-67.

Prentice, A. M.; Roberts, Susan B.; Watkinson, M.; Whitehead, Roger G.; Paul, Allison A.; Prentice, Ann; and Watkinson, Anne A. 1980. "Dietary Supplementation of Gambian Nursing Mothers and Lactational Performance." The Lancet 2 (October 25): 886-88.

Prentice, Ann; Prentice, A. M.; and Whitehead, Roger G. 1981. "Breast-Milk Fat Concentrations of Rural African Women. 2. Long-Term Variations within a Community." British Journal of Nutrition 45: 495-503.

Preston, Samuel H. 1979. "Urban Growth in Developing Countries: A Demographic Reappraisal." Population and Development Review 4: 195-215.

Prior, I. A. M. and Evans, J. Grimley. 1969. "Sodium Intake and Blood Pressure in Pacific Populations." Israel Journal of Medical Sciences 5: 608-11.

Quinn, Naomi. 1977. "Anthropological Studies on Women's Status." Annual Review of Anthropology 6: 181-225.

Rajalakshmi, R.; Subbulakshmi, G.; and Kotheri, B. 1974. "Ascorbic Acid Metabolism During Pregnancy and Lactation." Baroda Journal of Nutrition 1: 117.

Rakoff, A. E. 1968. "Endocrine Mechanisms in Psychogenic Amenorrhea." In Endocrinology and Human Behaviour: Proceedings of a Conference Held at the Institute of Psychiatry, London, 9 to 11 May 1967, edited by Richard Phillip Michael. London: Oxford University Press, pp. 139-60.

Rao, Kamala S. Jaya. 1979. "Attitudes to Women and Nutrition Programmes in India." The Lancet 2 (December 22/29): 1357-58.

Rao, Kamala S. Jaya; Mukherjee, N. R.; and Rao, K. Visweswana. 1972.

"A Survey of Diabetes Mellitus in a Rural Population of India." Diabetes 21: 1192-96.

Rao, N. P. and Vijayaraghavan, K. 1976. "Spin-off Benefits in Nutrition Programmes." Indian Journal of Medical Research 64: 1107-18.

Rao, Visweswana and Gopalan, C. 1971. "Family Size and Nutritional Status." In Report of the Workshop on Family Health. New Delhi: Population Council of India.

Reinhardt, Michaël C. 1978. "Maternal Anaemia in Abidjan--Its Influence on Placenta and Newborns." Helvetica Paediatrica Acta Suppl. 41: 43-63.

Remy, Dorothy. 1975. "Underdevelopment and the Experience of Women: A Nigerian Case Study." In Toward an Anthropology of Women, edited by Rayna R. Reiter. New York: Monthly Review Press, pp. 358-71.

Retel-Laurentin, Anne and Benoit, Daniel. 1976. "Infant Mortality and Birth Intervals." Population Studies 30: 279-93.

Reutlinger, Shlomo and Selowsky, Marcelo. 1976. "Malnutrition and Poverty: Magnitude and Policy Options." World Bank Occasional Papers, no. 23. Baltimore, MD: Johns Hopkins University Press.

Richards, Audrey Isabel. 1939. Land, Labor and Diet in Northern Rhodesia: An Economic Study of the Bemba Tribe. London: Oxford University for the International Institute of African Languages and Cultures.

_____ 1948. Hunger and Work in a Savage Tribe: A Functional Study of Nutrition Among the Southern Bantu. Glencoe, IL: The Free Press.

Ringrose, Helen and Zimmet, Paul. 1979. "Nutrient Intakes in an Urbanized Micronesian Population with a High Diabetes Prevalence." American Journal of Clinical Nutrition 32: 1334-41.

Rivera, M. Cecelia. 1979. "Labor Force Participation and Day Care Utilization by Low-Income Mothers in Bogotá, Colombia." Ph.D. dissertation, Brandeis University.

Robinson, John P.; Converse, Philip E., Jr.; and Szalai, Alexander. 1973. "Everyday Life in Twelve Countries." In The Use of Time: Daily Activities of Urban and Suburban Populations in Twelve Countries, edited by Alexander Szalai in collaboration with Philip E. Converse, Jr., Pierre Feldheim, Erwin K. Scheuch, and Philip J. Stone. The Hague: Mouton, pp. 113-44.

Rogers, Beatrice Lorge; Overholt, Catherine A.; Kennedy, Eileen; Sanchez, Federico; Chávez, Adolfo; Belding, Thomas K.; Timmer, C. Peter; and Austin, James E. 1981. Nutrition Intervention in Developing Countries. Vol. 4. Study V: Consumer Food Price Subsidies. Cambridge, MA: Oelgeschlager, Gunn & Hain.

Rogers, Everette M. and Kincaid, D. Lawrence. 1980. Communication Networks. Towards a New Paradigm for Research. New York: Free Press.

Rohde, Jon Eliot. 1978. "Preparing for the Next Round: Convalescent Care After Acute Infection." American Journal of Clinical Nutrition 31: 2248-68.

Rosaldo, Michele Zimbalist and Lamphere, Louise. 1974. Woman, Culture and Society. Stanford, CA: Stanford University Press.

Rosenberg, Irwin H.; Solomons, Noel W.; and Levin, Douglas M. 1976. "Interaction of Infection and Nutrition: Some Practical Concerns." Ecology of Food and Nutrition 4: 203-06.

Rowland, M. G. M.; Paul, Alison A.; Prentice, A. M.; Muller, Elisabeth; Hutton, Melanie; Barrell, R. A. E.; and Whitehead, Roger G. 1981. "Seasonality and the Growth of Infants in a Gambian Village." In Seasonal Dimensions to Rural Poverty, edited by Robert Chambers, Richard Longhurst, and Arnold Pacey. London: Pinter; Totowa, NJ: Allanheld, Osmun, pp. 164-75.

Rush, David; Stein, Zena; and Sussner, Mervyn. 1980. Diet in Pregnancy: A Randomized Controlled Trial of Prenatal Nutritional

Supplementation. Birth Defects: Original Article Series, Vol. 16, no. 3. New York: Alan R. Liss.

Russell, Marcia. 1976. "The Relationship of Family Size and Spacing to Growth of Preschool Mayan Children in Guatemala." American Journal of Public Health 66: 1165-72.

Rutherford, R. S. 1975. "The Influence of Child Mortality on Fertility: A Review of Mechanisms." In Seminar on Infant Mortality in Relation to the Level of Fertility. Bangkok, Thailand: Comité International de Coordination des Recherches Nationales en Démographie.

Sacks, Karen. 1970. "Social Bases for Sexual Equality: A Comparative View." In Sisterhood Is Powerful: An Anthology of Writings from the Women's Liberation Movement, edited by Robin Morgan. New York: Random House, pp. 455-69.

Saffioti, H. I. B. 1975. "Female Labor and Capitalism in the U.S. and Brazil." In Women Cross-Culturally: Challenge and Change, edited by Ruby Rohrlich-Leavitt. World Anthropology Series. The Hague: Mouton.

Safilios-Rothschild, Constantina. 1980. "The Role of the Family: A Neglected Aspect of Poverty." Background paper, World Development Report. Washington, DC: International Bank for Reconstruction and Development.

Sakr, E. 1973. The Effect of Contraceptive Steroids on Bilharzial Liver. Cairo: Al Azhar University.

Satyanarayana, K. and Naidu, A. Nadamuni. 1979. "Nutrition and Menarche in Rural Hyderabad." Annals of Human Biology 6: 163-65.

Satyanarayana, K.; Hanumantha, D.; Rao, D. H.; Rao, D. V.; and Swaminathan, M. 1972. "Nutrition and Working Efficiency in Coal-miners." Indian Journal of Medical Research 60: 1800-06.

Schofield, Sue. 1979. Development and the Problems of Village Nutrition. Montclair, NJ: Allanheld, Osmun in association with the Institute of Development Studies, Sussex.

Schultz, Theodore W. 1975. "The Value of the Ability to Deal with Disequilibria." Journal of Economic Literature 13: 827-46.

Schultz, Yves; Lechtig, Aaron; and Bradfield, Robert B. 1980. "Energy Expenditure and Food Intakes of Lactating Women in Guatemala." American Journal of Clinical Nutrition 33: 892-902.

Scragg, Roy F. R. 1973. "Menopause and Reproductive Life Span in Rural New Guinea." Paper presented to the Annual Symposium of the Papua New Guinea Medical Society, Port Moresby.

Scrimshaw, Nevin S. 1975. "Interactions of Malnutrition and Infection: Advances in Understanding." In Protein-Calorie Malnutrition, edited by Robert E. Olson. Nutrition Foundation Monograph Series. San Francisco: Academic Press.

_____. 1980. "A Look at the Incaparina Experience in Guatemala: The Background and History of Incaparina." Food and Nutrition Bulletin 2 (2): 1-2.

Scrimshaw, Neven S.; Taylor, Carl E.; and Gordon, John E. 1966. Interactions of Nutrition and Infection. WHO Monograph Series, no. 57. Geneva: World Health Organization.

Seftel, H. C. 1978. "The Rarity of Coronary Heart Disease in South African Blacks." South African Medical Journal 54: 99-105.

Selowsky, Marcelo and Taylor, Lance. 1973. "The Economics of Malnourished Children: An Example of Disinvestment in Human Capital." Economic Development and Cultural Change 22: 17-30.

Sever, P. S.; Peart, W. S.; Gordon, D.; and Beighton, P. 1980. "Blood Pressure and Its Correlates in Urban and Tribal Africa." The Lancet 2 (July 12): 60-64.

Shah, P. M. 1977. The Kasa MCHN Project--The Third Progress Report. Bombay: CARE.

Shaper, A. G. 1972. "Cardiovascular Disease in the Tropics--IV. Coronary Heart Disease." British Medical Journal 4: 32-35.

Sharman, Anne. 1970. "Nutrition and Social Planning." Journal of Development Studies 6 (4): 77-91.

Shiffman, Morris A.; Schneider, R.; Faigenblum, Jacques M.; Helms, Ronald W.; and Turner, Alvis G. 1978. "Field Studies on Water Sanitation and Health Education in Relation to Health Status in Central America." Progress in Water Technology 11: 143-50.

Shirai, Yoichi and Matsuo, Takehumi. 1967. "Epidemiological Study of Hypertension in Relation to Nutritional State of Indonesian People." Kobe Journal of Medicine 13: 165-69.

Simmons, Ozzie G. 1981. "Population and Integrated Programs." Prepared as an introductory overview for sessions on "Integrated Approaches in Population: Information Resources," Association for Population/Family Planning Libraries and Information Centers--International, 14th Annual Conference, Washington, DC, March 23-26.

Simpson, I. A. and Chow, A. Y. 1956. "The Thiamine Content of Human Milk in Malaya. Part I. The 'Normal' Level of Thiamine in Milk from Malay, Chinese and Indian Women." Journal of Tropical Pediatrics 2: 3-17.

Singarimbun, Masri and Manning, Chris. 1976. "Breastfeeding, Amenorrhea, and Abstinence in a Javanese Village: A Case Study of Mojolama." Studies in Family Planning 7: 175-79.

Singh, Andrea Menefee. 1977. "Women and the Family: Coping with Poverty in the Bastis of Delhi." Social Action 27: 257-59.

Sinha, Dinesh P. 1980. "Overnutrition and Related Diseases (Diabetes and Cardiovascular Diseases): A Major Public Health Problem in the English-speaking Caribbean. A Position Paper." Kingston, Jamaica: Caribbean Food and Nutrition Institute and Pan American Health Organization, Pan American Sanitary Bureau, Regional Office of the World Health Organization.

Sogbanmu, M. O. and Aregbesola, Y. A. 1979. "Menarchal Age in Nigerian School-girls: Its Relationship to Their Height, Weight and Menstrual Profile." International Journal of Gynecology and Obstetrics 16: 339-40.

Solomons, Noel W. and Keusch, Gerald T. 1981. "Nutritional Implications of Parasitic Infections." Nutrition Reviews 39: 149-61.

Solon, Florentino S.; Popkin, Barry M.; Fernandez, Thomas L.; and Latham, Michael C. 1978. "Vitamin A Deficiency in the Philippines: A Study of Xerophthalmia in Cebu." American Journal of Clinical Nutrition 31: 360-68.

Soukupova, Kveta and Prusova, Felicitas. 1970. "Nutrition and the Ischemic Heart Disease Mortality Rates in 33 Countries." Nutrition and Metabolism 12: 240-44.

Soysa, Piyani E. and Jayasuriya, Devika S. 1975. "Birth Weight in Ceylonese." Human Biology 47: 1-15.

Spellacy, William N. 1974. "Metabolic Effects of Oral Contraceptives." Clinical Obstetrics and Gynecology 1 (1): 53-64.

Stanley, Joyce with Lundeen, Alison. 1978. "Audio Cassette Listening Forums: A Participatory Women's Development Project." Prepared for Women in Development, U.S. Agency for International Development. Washington, DC.

Stein, Zena; Susser, Mervyn; and Rush, David. 1978. "Prenatal Nutrition and Birth Weight: Experiments and Quasi-Experiments in the Past Decade." Journal of Reproductive Medicine 21: 287-99.

Stein, Zena; Susser, Mervyn; Saenger, Gerhart; and Marolla, Francis. 1975. Famine and Human Development: The Dutch Hunger Winter 1944-1945. London: Oxford University Press.

Stoler, Ann. 1977. "Class Structure and Female Autonomy in Rural Java." Signs 3: 74-89.

Stuart, J. E. and Connellan, P. 1973. "Ascorbic Acid Studies in Aborigines." Australian Paediatric Journal 9: 159-63.

Sukhatme, P. V. 1977. "Malnutrition and Poverty." Ninth Lal Bahaduri Shastri Memorial Lecture, Indian Agricultural Research Institute, New Delhi.

Sundararaj, Regina and Pereira, Sheila M. 1975. "Dietary Intakes and Food Taboos of Lactating Women in a South Indian Community." Tropical and Geographical Medicine 27: 189-93.

Susser, Mervyn. 1981. "Prenatal Nutrition, Birth Weight, and Psychological Development: An Overview of Experiments, Quasi-experiments, and Natural Experiments in the Past Decade." American Journal of Clinical Nutrition 34: 784-803.

Taffel, Selma. 1978. Prenatal Care, United States, 1969-75. Vital and Health Statistics: Series 21, Data from the National Vital Statistics System, no. 33. DHEW Publication no. (PHS) 78-1911. Hyattsville, MD: National Center for Health Statistics; Public Health Service; Department of Health, Education, and Welfare.

Tandberg, A. 1980. "Summer Project 1980: Final Report on the Participation in the Implementation of the Mass Media Nutrition Project in Kinshasa." New Orleans: Nutrition Department, Tulane University.

Tanner, J. M. 1968. "Earlier Maturation in Man." Scientific American 218: 21-27.

Taylor, C. Bruce and Ho, Kang-Jey. 1971. "Studies on the Masai." American Journal of Clinical Nutrition 24: 1291-93.

Taylor, Lance; Horton, Susan; and Roff, Daniel. 1980. "Food Subsidy Programs: A Survey." Cambridge, MA: Massachusetts Institute of Technology.

Thanangkul, Ousa and Amatayakul, Kosin. 1975. "Nutrition of Pregnant Women in a Developing Country--Thailand." American Journal of Diseases of Children 129: 426-27.

Theuer, Richard C. 1972. "Effect of Oral Contraceptive Agents on Vitamin and Mineral Needs: A Review." Journal of Reproductive Medicine 8: 13-19.

Thomson, Angus M. 1959. "Maternal Stature and Reproductive Efficiency." Eugenics Review 51: 157-62.

Thomson, Angus M. and Billewicz, W. Z. 1975. "Nutritional Status, Maternal Physique and Reproductive Efficiency." Proceedings of the Nutrition Society 22: 55-60.

Thomson, Angus M. and Black A. E. 1975. "Nutritional Aspects of Human Lactation." Bulletin of the World Health Organization 52: 163-77.

Thomson, Angus M. and Hytten, Frank E. 1978. "Nutrition During Pregnancy." In Nutrition and the World Food Problem, edited by Miloslav Rechigl, Jr. Basel: Karger.

Thomson, Angus M.; Beaton, George H.; Habicht, Jean-Pierre; and Underwood, Barbara A. 1979. "Nutrition During Pregnancy: A Review." Paper prepared for the ACC Sub-Committee on Nutrition, Consultative Group on Maternal and Young Child Nutrition, Rome, November 5-7.

Thomson, Angus M.; Billewicz, W. Z.; and Hytten, Frank E. 1968. "The Assessment of Fetal Growth." Journal of Obstetrics and Gynaecology of the British Commonwealth 75: 903-16.

Thomson, Angus M.; Billewicz, W. Z.; Thompson, Barbara; and McGregor, I. A. 1966. "Body Weight Changes During Pregnancy and Lactation in Rural African (Gambian) Women." Journal of Obstetrics and Gynaecology of the British Commonwealth 73: 724-33.

Tietze, Christopher. 1968. "Fertility After Discontinuation of Intrauterine and Oral Contraception." International Journal of Fertility 13: 385-89.

Tindal, J. S. 1974. "Hypothalamic Control of Secretion and Release of Prolactin." Journal of Reproduction and Fertility 39: 437-61.

Tinker, Irene. 1976. "Development and the Disintegration of the Family." Les Carnets de l'enface 36: 37.

_____ 1979. "New Technologies for Food Chain Activities: The Imperative of Equity for Women." Washington, DC: Office of Women in Development, U.S. Agency for International Development.

Tompkins, Winslow T.; Wiehl, Dorothy G.; and Mitchell, Robert McN. 1955. "The Underweight Patient as an Increased Obstetric Hazard." American Journal of Obstetrics and Gynecology 69: 114-23.

Trussell, James. 1980. "Statistical Flaws in Evidence for the Frisch Hypothesis that Fatness Triggers Menarche." Human Biology 52: 711-20.

Tyson, John E. and Perez, Alfredo. 1978. "The Maintenance of Infecundity in Postpartum Women." In Nutrition and Human Reproduction, edited by W. Henry Mosley. New York: Plenum, pp. 11-28.

Underwood, Barbara A. 1981. "Marginal Malnutrition and Reproductive Performance." Paper presented to the XII International Congress of Nutrition, San Diego, CA, August 16-21.

UN. See United Nations

United Nations. 1975. Selected World Demographic Indicators by Country, 1950-2000. ESA/P/WP.55. New York: Department of Economic and Social Affairs, United Nations.

_____ 1979a. Demographic Estimates and Projections for the World, Regions and Countries Assessed in 1978. Provisional report. New York: Department of International Economic and Social Affairs, United Nations.

_____ 1979b. An Integrated Approach to Population, Food and Nutrition Policies and Programs for National Development. Asian Population Studies Series, no. 45. Bangkok.

_____ 1980. Development Forum 7 (5). [United Nations University and the Division of Economic and Social Information/DPI.] United States. Agency for International Development, Technical Assistance Bureau, Office of Nutrition (1976) Application of a Field Guide for Evaluation of Nutrition Education in Three Programs in Brazil. Washington, DC.

USAID. See United States. Agency for International Development.

Valdecañas, Ofelia C. 1971. "Barrio Central: A Study of Some Social and Cultural Factors in Malnutrition." Philippine Journal of Nutrition 24: 223-37.

Valenzuela, Rosario E. 1978. "A Study on Nutrient Distribution Within the Family and Factors Affecting Nutrient Intake." Philippine Economic Journal 36: 168-84.

Valenzuela, Rosario E.; Florencio, Cecilia; and Guthrie, Helen. 1979. "Distribution of Nutrients Within the Filipino Family." Nutrition Reports International 19: 573-81.

Valverde, Victor; Delgado, Hernán L.; Hurtado, Elena; and Klein, Robert E. 1981. "Maternal Weight Changes and Energy Intake During Pregnancy and Lactation." Paper presented to the XII International Congress of Nutrition, San Diego, CA, August 16-21.

van den Berg, Bea J. 1977. "Epidemiologic Observations of Prematurity: Effects of Tobacco, Coffee, and Alcohol." In The Epidemiology of Pregnancy, edited by Dwayne M. Reed and Fiona J. Stanley. Baltimore: Urban & Schwarzenberg, pp. 157-76.

Van Ginneken, Jeroen K. 1978. "The Impact of Prolonged Breast Feeding on Birth Intervals and on Postpartum Amenorrhea." In Nutrition and Human Reproduction, edited by W. Henry Mosley. New York: Plenum, pp. 179-96.

Van Itallie, Theodore B. 1979. "Obesity: Adverse Effects on Health and Longevity." American Journal of Clinical Nutrition 32: 2723-33.

van 't Hof, Martin A. and Roede, Machteld J. 1977. "A Monte Carlo Test of Weight as a Critical Factor in Menarche, Compared with Bone

Age and Measures of Height, Width, and Sexual Development." Annals of Human Biology 4: 581-85.

Venkatachalam, P.S. 1962. A Study of Diet, Nutrition, and Health of the People of the Chimbu Area, New Guinea Highlands. Monograph no. 4. Port Moresby: Department of Public Health, Territories of Papua New Guinea.

_____ 1968. "Iron Metabolism and Iron Deficiency in India." American Journal of Clinical Nutrition 21: 1156-61.

Venkatachalam, P. S.; Shankar, K.; and Gopalan, C. 1960. "Changes in Body-Weight and Body Composition During Pregnancy." Indian Journal of Medical Research 48: 511-17.

Villa-Real, Romulo. 1975. "Breast Feeding in the Philippines, a Benefit-Cost Analysis." Quezon City: School of Economics, University of the Philippines.

Vitalis, P. 1980. "Nutrition Education in a Family Planning Clinic." Health Education Bulletin, no. 17. Rockwell, MD: National Clearinghouse for Family Planning Information.

Viteri, Fernando E. 1971. "Considerations on the Effect of Nutrition on the Body Composition and Physical Working Capacity of Young Guatemalan Adults." In Amino Acid Fortification of Protein Foods; Report of an International Conference Held at the Massachusetts Institute of Technology, September 16 to 18, 1969, edited by Nevin S. Scrimshaw and Aaron M. Altschul. Cambridge, MA: MIT Press, pp. 350-75.

_____ 1976. "Definition of the Nutrition Problem in the Labor Force." In Nutrition and Agricultural Development, edited by Nevin S. Scrimshaw and Mois'Se B'Ehar. Basic Life Science Series, vol. 7. New York: Plenum.

Vouri, E.; Kiuru, K.; Mäkinen, S. M.; Väyrynen, P.; Kara, R.; and Kuitunen, P. 1982. "Maternal Diet and Fatty Acid Pattern of Breast Milk." Acta Paediatrica Scandivica 71: 959-63.

Warren, Michelle P. 1973. "Metabolic Effects of Contraceptive Steroids." American Journal of the Medical Sciences 265: 5-21.

Welch, Finis. 1973. "The Role of Investments in Human Capital in Agriculture." In Distortions of Agricultural Incentives, edited by Theodore William Schultz. Bloomington: Indiana University Press, pp. 259-81.

_____ 1970. "Education in Production." Journal of Political Economy 78: 35-59.

West, Kelly M. and Kalbfleisch, John M. 1966. "Glucose Tolerance, Nutrition, and Diabetes in Uruguay, Venezuela, Malaya, and East Pakistan." Diabetes 15: 9-18.

_____ 1970. "Diabetes in Central America." Diabetes 19: 656-63.

_____ 1971. "Influence of Nutritional Factors on Prevalence of Diabetes." Diabetes 20: 99-108.

Whichelow, Margaret J. 1975. "Calorie Requirements for Successful Breast Feeding." Archives of Diseases in Childhood 50: 669.

_____ 1976. "Success and Failure of Breast-feeding in Relation to Energy Intake." Proceedings of the Nutrition Society 35 (2): 62A-63A.

Whitehead, Floy E. 1970. Nutrition Education Research Project-- Report of Feasibility Study. Washington, DC: Office of Nutrition, Technical Assistance Bureau, U.S. Agency for International Development.

Whitehead, Roger G. 1980. "The Better Use of Food Resources for Infants and Mothers." Proceedings of the Royal Society of London, Series B 209: 59-69.

Whitehead, Roger G.; Rowland, M. G. M.; Hutton, Melanie; Prentice, A. M.; Müller, Elisabeth; and Paul, Alison A. 1978. "Factors Influencing Lactation Performance in Rural Gambian Mothers." The Lancet 2 (July 22): 178-81.

WHO. See World Health Organization.

Whyte, Robert Orr and White, Pauline. 1978. Rural Asian Women: Status and Environment. Research Notes and Discussion paper, no. 9. Singapore: Institute of Southeast Asian Studies.

Wilmsen, Edwin N. 1978. "Seasonal Effects of Dietary Intake on Kalahari San." Federation Proceedings 37, no. 1, "Anthropology and the Assessment of Nutritional Status," pp. 65-72.

Wilson, Christine S. 1978. "Food Taboos at Childbirth: The Malay Example." Ecology of Food and Nutrition 2: 267-74.

Winikoff, Beverly. 1978. "Nutrition, Population, and Health: Some implications for Policy." Science 200 (May 26): 895-902.

Wishik, Samuel M. 1977. "The Implications of Undernutrition During Pubescence and Adolescence on Fertility." In Nutritional Impacts on Women Throughout Life with Emphasis on Reproduction, edited by Kamran S. Moghissi and Tommy N. Evans. Hagerstown, MD: Harper & Row, pp. 23-24.

Wishik, Samuel M. and Van der Vynkt, Susan. 1975. "Nutrition, Mother's Health and Fertility: The Effects of Childbearing on Health and Nutrition." PAG Bulletin 5 (3): 11-17.

Wolfe, Barbara L.; Behrman, Jere R.; Belli, Humberto; Cairns, Kathleen; and Williamson, Nancy. 1980. "Socioeconomic Characteristics of Women in a Developing Country and the Degree of Urbanization." Institute for Research on Poverty Discussion Paper, no. 655-81. Madison: University of Wisconsin-Madison.

Woods, William G.; Mills, Elaine; and Ferrieri, Patricia. 1974. "Neonatal Malaria Due to Plasmodium Vivax." Journal of Pediatrics 84: 669-71.

World Bank. 1979. Recognizing the "Invisible" Woman in Development: The World Bank's Experience. Washington, DC.

World Health Organization. 1970a. Nutritional Status of Populations: A Manual on Anthropometric Appraisal of Trends. NUTR/70.129.

_____. 1970b. Spontaneous and Induced Abortion. Report of a WHO Scientific Group. Technical Report Series, no. 461. Geneva.

_____. 1972. "Nutrition: A Review of the WHO Programme, 1965-1971." WHO Chronicle 26: 160-95.

_____. 1973. Advances in Methods of Fertility Regulation. Report of a WHO Scientific Group. Technical Report Series, no. 527. Geneva.

_____. 1975. The Epidemiology of Infertility. Technical Report Series, no. 582. Geneva.

_____. 1979. The Prevalence of Nutritional Anaemia in Women in Developing Countries. Geneva.

_____. 1980a. Health and the Status of Women. FHE/80.1. Geneva.

_____. 1980b. "The Incidence of Low Birth Weight: A Critical Review of Available Information." World Health Statistics Quarterly 33: 197-224.

_____. 1980c. World Health Statistics. Vol. 1. Vital Statistics and Cause of Death. Geneva.

_____. 1980d. "Report of the Second Scientific Working Group in Social and Economic Research: Guidelines to Assess the Social and Economic Consequences of the Tropical Diseases." Draft. Geneva.

Wray, Joe D. 1971. "Population Pressure on Families: Family Size and Child Spacing." In Rapid Population Growth: Consequences and Policy Implications, prepared by a Study Committee of the Office of the Foreign Secretary, National Academy of Sciences with the support of the Agency for International Development. Baltimore: Johns Hopkins Press for the National Academy of Sciences, pp. 403-61.

_____. 1978. "Maternal Nutrition, Breast-feeding and Infant Survival." In Nutrition and Human Reproduction, edited by W. Henry Mosley. New York: Plenum, pp. 197-230.

Wray, Joe D. and Aguirre, Alfredo. 1969. "Protein-Calorie Malnutrition in Candelaria, Colombia. I. Prevalence; Social and Demographic Causal Factors." Journal of Tropical Pediatrics 15: 76-98.

Wyon, John B.; Finner, Stephen L.; and Gordon, John E. 1966. "Differential Age at Menopause in Rural Punjab, India." Population Index 32: 328.

Youssef, Nadia Haggag. 1974. Women and Work in Developing Societies. Population Monograph Series, no. 15. Westport, CT: Greenwood Press.

Zacharias, Leona W. and Wurtman, Richard J. 1969. "Age at Menarche: Genetic and Environmental Influences." New England Journal of Medicine 280 (April 17): 868-75.

Zacharias, Leona W.; Rand, William M.; and Wurtman, Richard J. 1976. "A Prospective Study of Sexual Development and Growth in American Girls: The Statistics of Menarche." Obstetrical and Gynecological Survey 31: 325-37.

Zeitlin, Marian F. and Formacion, Candelaria S. 1981. Nutrition Intervention in Developing Countries. Vol. 2. Study II. Nutrition Education. Cambridge, MA: Oelgeschlager, Gunn & Hain.

Zeitlin, Marian F.; Schlossman, Nina; Meurer, Michael; Wray, Joe D.; and Stanbury, John. 1980. "Nutrition-Fertility Interactions in Developing Countries: Implications for Program Design." Paper prepared for the Office of Policy Development and Program Review, Agency for International Development. Washington, DC.

Zeitlin, Marian F.; Wray, Joe D.; Stanburg, John B.; Schlossman, Nina P.; Meurer, Michael J.; and Wienthal, Patricia J. 1982. Nutrition and Population. The Delicate Balance. Cambridge, MA: Oelgeschlager, Gunn & Hain.

Zimmet, Paul. 1979. "Epidemiology of Diabetes and Its Macrovascular Manifestations in Pacific Populations: The Medical Effects of Social Progress." Diabetes Care 2: 144-53.

INDEX

Afghanistan, 15

Africa, 14, 16, 19, 26, 31, 39, 41, 42, 45, 47, 49, 50, 52
    See also specific countries

Agriculture: extension and nutrition-family planning cooperation, 76; productivity and development programs, 77-78; work, effect on child care in Malaysia, 40

Amenorrhea: and malnutrition, 8-9

Amenorrhea, lactational: 9-11; and body fat, 9, 10 (in Bangladesh, 10, 11; Gambia, 10; Guatemala, 10, 11; India, 10; Mexico, 11)

Anemia: among women, 15-16, 21, 31, 55; and IUD use, 34, 81; and labor productivity (in Guatemala, 21; Sri Lanka, 20-21); and malaria, 31; and spontaneous abortion, 34; defined, 15

"Appropriate technologies": 79

Asia, 14, 16, 26, 39, 47, 49, 50, 52
    See also specific countries

Assets, household: effects on nutrition, 36

Bangladesh, 6, 7, 10, 11, 13, 15, 38, 45, 52

Belgium, 14

Birth weight: as infant health status indicator, 4; effects of mother's pre-pregnancy size on in Guatemala, 6; increased through maternal supplements, 4

Birth weight, low: as proxy for maternal nutrition status, 25; defined, 4; prevalence of, 5, 25-26 (in Kenya, 5; Africa, Asia, Latin America, 26); statistical problems, 25

Botswana, 38

Brazil, 24, 35

Breast milk: as best for infants, 66; composition, 14; dietary intake needed to produce, 33; fat content, 13; protein content, 13-14; quality, 13-14 (in Bangladesh, 13; Belgium, 14; Gambia, 13; Japan, 14; Peru, 13; Sweden, 14); quantity, 12-13 (in Gambia, 12-13; Great Britain, 12); volume, 10

Breast-feeding: and amenorrhea, 9-11; promotion of, 74
    See also breast milk; lactation

Bureau of Agricultural Extension (Philippines): and family planning, 76

Calories. See energy

Cameroon, 36

Caribbean, 19, 42, 50
    See also specific countries

Cash cropping: 77, 78, 79

Ceylon, 19

Child care: and mother's nutrition, 21; by mother substitutes, 41-42; effect of mother's work on, 39, 40; seasonal variations in, 44

Children: as focus of nutrition intervention programs, 59, 60, 62

Chile, 15

China, 29

Cholesterol levels: and coronary heart disease, 19

Colombia, 4, 41, 62, 64, 67

Contraceptives, use of: and social networks in Korea, 53; effects on women's nutrition, 34-35, 74, 81; hormonal, 34-35 (in Egypt, 35); and lactation suppression, 35; IUD, 34

Cultural preferences: and policy, 84; and women's status, 43, 53; for food, 52; for obesity, 52

Deaths. See mortality

Deficiencies, dietary: amenable to food fortification, 71; and disease, 16, 17, 31

Development programs: and women's nutritional status, 77-79, 83, 85 (in Kenya, 78); as aid to overcoming seasonal problems, 83; relationship to fertility, 78

Diabetes mellitus, 18-19

Dietary recommendations: WHO, 23

Disease, 15-20; and parity, 42; chronic, 17-20; infectious, 16-17, 30-31, 81; nutritional deficiency, 16, 17, 31; relationship to hormonal contraceptive use, 35; relationship to nutrition, 30-32

Diseases "of affluence," 17-20

Economic value of family members, 37, 52

Ecuador, 66

Education: and policy, 84; disparities by sex, 50, 78; effects on nutrition, 49-50, 57; effects on women, 50; opportunities for women, 50 (in Africa, Asia, Caribbean, Middle East, Latin America, 50)
    See also nutrition education programs

Egypt, 24, 35